Chairman
S. R. HIRSCH

Psychiatric Beds and Resources: Factors Influencing Bed Use and Service Planning

Report of a Working Party of the Section for Social and Community Psychiatry of the Royal College of Psychiatrists

The Royal College of Psychiatrists is grateful to The Priory Hospital, London SW15, *for meeting the cost of printing this report*

GASKELL

Contents

Members and observers of the Bed Norms and Resources Working Party

Professor S. R. Hirsch (Chairman), Section for Social and Community Psychiatry, Royal College of Psychiatrists

Mr B. Gerrard, Research Section, London Borough of Ealing Social Services

Mr H. Malin, Operational Research Section, Department of Health and Social Services

Dr A. Brown, Section for Social and Community Psychiatry, Royal College of Psychiatrists

Dr T. Fryers, Department of Community Medicine, University of Manchester

Dr D. Dick, Previously Director, Health Advisory Service, and Royal College of Psychiatrists

Dr C. Jennings, Psychiatric Case Register Group

Dr A Baker, Health Advisory Service (visitor)

Dr T. P. Riordan, Health Advisory Service (visitor)

Dr P. Rogers, Health Advisory Service (visitor)

Dr A. Sippert, Department of Health and Social Services (observer)

Mrs P. Williamson, Department of Health and Social Services (observer)

Mr Chan Himatsingani, Department of Health and Social Services (observer)

Dr P. W. Brooks, Scottish Home and Health Department

When originally constituted, members of the Working Party included Drs H. L. Freeman, J. Grimshaw, P. Jefferys, H. Mair, P. Mason and U. Seidel. J. Yates contributed on one occasion, and Drs B. Robinson, G. Ooman, and S. Martin assisted in the collection of data.

Preface

The Working Party on Bed Norms and Resources of the Section for Social and Community Psychiatry of the Royal College of Psychiatrists was established in 1978 to make recommendations to planners about bed norms for district psychiatric services. The working party started by examining the guidelines for bed provision for the acutely mentally ill adult under 65 years of age. The first report (Hirsch, 1983), with a detailed statement of aims, discussed the concept of a norm and the factors which might affect numbers of beds and their use; the remit was to look at the Department of Health and Social Security (DHSS) district general-hospital (DGH)-based norm. The working party used a variety of approaches, including on-site visits to a sample of hospitals; the sample was slanted towards DGH-based services. What emerged was that beds, whether located in a DGH or in a mental hospital, are only one component of a service. Whether the allocation of locally available resources should be slanted towards beds and other services within the hospital, or towards community resources, and whether the beds provided should be based in a DGH or in an acute-case unit in a mental hospital, are mainly matters for local decision. However, beds in acute-case units, with their need for nursing and other support services, form the most expensive nodal point of a service, and their consideration is therefore a useful starting point for a study of the resources needed for a district-based service.

Although the working party did not concern itself with the question of patients requiring long-term hospital care, clearly it must not be overlooked. The accumulation of one patient a year, with a life expectancy of 40 years, will eventually keep 40 beds filled indefinitely, and five new chronically ill patients per year will eventually require 200 beds. It follows that although this report is concerned with resource planning for acute-case services, the planning for rehabilitation may, after 10 years, be more important than planning for acute-case beds.

The working party did not seek to provide an exhaustive explanation of why some district services have more resources than others. Its main concern was to examine the other elements of a service which affect bed provision and bed use, and to offer an approach to analysing these aspects, but without prescriptions as to how services should be organised. This is a constantly developing issue. It is primarily up to the local clinicians and planners, informed by the views of consumers in the local community, to decide what kind of therapeutic team is wanted, how best to organise the service, and what particular resources are to be increased or diminished.

The working party's concern was therefore to provide a method of estimating the amount of resources needed: beds are only one element of this, but, given present practice, they play a central part. Once it has been decided whether certain resources need to be increased or diminished, decisions can then be taken which may shift the emphasis from intramural to day or domiciliary services. It is hoped that this report will shed useful light on that process.

The report includes both a review of the literature and some important new data; these show a close relationship between social factors and the uptake of psychiatric services, as well as the prevalence of psychiatric disorder (see chapter 2). This should be helpful to planners in predicting the likely level of psychiatric requirements in a particular catchment-area population. A study carried out with the co-operation of the Psychiatric Case Register Group enabled the working party to look at bed use (in contrast to bed provision) by the populations which were being monitored by registers in seven areas in the UK (chapter 3). There is also a description of the working party's study of 20 DGH-based psychiatric services, chosen from regional health authorities throughout England and Wales. This includes an analysis of 400 discharges in the same year at each hospital (chapter 4), and one analysis of current bed provision and use in the 20 hospitals studied, as compared with case-register and national figures (chapter 5).

The working party took a detailed look at service policy, organisation, and support services to determine the contribution they make to the three-fold variation in bed/population ratios among the 20 hospitals studied (chapter 6). Chapter 7 demonstrates an approach to psychiatric planning which is based on an analysis of service provision, utilisation, and potential demand, drawn from the information established earlier. Chapter 8 makes recommendations for planners based on the findings. Each chapter has a summary, and the overall findings are briefly summarised in chapter 9.

Acknowledgements

The working party is indebted to many colleagues who participated in discussions and helped to collect and analyse the information on which the report is based. Mr H. Malin, of the DHSS Operational Research Section, helped prepare both the questionnaire and the background work for visits to the 20 hospitals. Mr B. Gerrard, of the Research Section of the London Borough of Ealing Social Services Department, undertook statistical analyses and the preparation of most of the tables in the report. Dr P. Brooks, of the Scottish Home and Health Department, acted as rapporteur at meetings, as well as collecting and helping to draft the review of the literature. His support, and that of Mr Gerrard and Mr Malin, was valuable in helping us to complete this exercise. Dr D. Dick formulated the concept of the elements of a comprehensive service, which provided a structure for the 20-hospital study; also when Director of the Health Advisory Service (HAS), he funded Dr S. Martin, who carried out the analysis of 400 discharged patients, and the on-site consultations carried out by the HAS visitors, Dr A. A. Baker, Dr T. P. Riordan, and Dr P. Rogers. The working party is grateful to Dr P. Horrocks (who succeeded Dr Dick as Director of the HAS) for continuing support. Mr C. Jennings, of the Psychiatric Case Register Group, did all the analysis of that study. Dr R. C. Driscoll performed the analysis of the variation in admission rates with indicators of underprivilege for the districts of the North West Thames Regional Health Authority, and made some revision of chapters 2 and 7. Dr B. Robinson and Dr G. Ooman carried out a pilot study. Professor S. R. Hirsch and Dr R. C. Driscoll co-authored Appendix 3.

The Chairman, who prepared this report, is indebted to all those colleagues, as well as to other members of the working party, who contributed ideas and comments, and scrutinised the manuscript. Thanks are due to Yvonne Kemp, Tricia Carroll, and Moira McKnight, who helped format and type the report through many drafts. Editing was carried out by Dr G. Wilkinson and Professor H. Freeman.

S. R. HIRSCH

1 Introduction

In the late 1970s, the Section for Social and Community Psychiatry of the Royal College of Psychiatrists set up a working party to reconsider Department of Health and Social Security (DHSS) guidelines on the number of beds required for acute-case psychiatric services. The wide variation in bed use between health districts, regional health authorities, and London boroughs, which had been noted over the previous ten years, suggested differences in practice, demand, or need for in-patient and psychiatric treatment. Table I shows the psychiatric beds per 1000 population in different regional health authorities in 1982, the latest year for which data were available. These figures give some indication of the problem. The DHSS 1971 circular (HM(71)97), and 1975 White Paper, *Better Services for the Mentally Ill*, recommended a single figure of 0.5 acute-case beds per 1000 population as the norm for district general-hospital (DGH)-based units, with no indication as to how authorities should estimate how their needs might vary from this norm.

Because health authorities had begun to adopt local planning figures, based on limited local experience, as their guidelines, the working party was set up to re-examine the problem, and to make recommendations that would assist planners in deciding bed requirements for acute-case psychiatry. It seemed likely that the concept of a single norm for this purpose should be replaced by an approach which would enable bed provisions to be varied according to local needs, as was the original DHSS intention. This norm was meant to be only a guideline, and came to be understood as referring to acutely ill patients admitted to DGH-based units, but excluding long-stay patients (whether new or established) after 1 year. It has been assumed that existing hospital provision could cater for patients with dementia, but in view of the rapidly increasing numbers of elderly patients, the guidelines were adjusted to allow an additional 0.65 beds per 1000 total over-65 population. Given the Government intention to provide more psychiatric beds for acute-case psychiatry at DGH sites, and to phase out mental-hospital-based services, the working party decided to limit its remit to acutely ill DGH-treated psychiatric patients staying in hospital for up to 1 year. Bed needs for long-stay patients, the elderly severely mentally infirm (ESMI), children, and adolescents were not considered.

The first report (Hirsch, 1983) should be read in conjunction with this present one. It was recognised that norms tend to reflect existing bed use, in terms of beds in actual use related to population, but that this only indicated the *average* level

TABLE I

Resident patients with mental illness in 1982, per 1000 population in different regions in England

Region	Acute (over 15 years) [length of stay less than 1 year]: admitted 1982	New long-stay patients admitted 1971–1981	Established long-stay patients admitted since 1970	Totals
Northern	0.60	0.63	0.44	1.67
Yorkshire	0.62	0.60	0.44	1.66
Trent	0.57	0.50	0.34	1.41
East Anglia	0.59	0.50	0.25	1.33
N W Thames	0.63	0.71	0.61	1.95
N E Thames	0.60	0.56	0.43	1.59
S E Thames	0.73	0.50	0.46	1.69
S W Thames	0.64	0.72	0.69	2.05
Wessex	0.54	0.48	0.24	1.26
Oxford	0.35	0.25	0.23	0.83
South Western	0.59	0.53	0.36	1.48
West Midlands	0.48	0.54	0.31	1.33
Mersey	0.76	0.84	0.56	2.17
North Western	0.58	0.49	0.44	1.51
England	0.59	0.56	0.41	1.56

The figures were supplied by Statistics Division, DHSS, from Mental Health Enquiry data, and indicate the psychiatric beds in use for acute-case, and both new and established long-stay, patients with mental illness (including psycho-geriatric patients). The population data are based on the 1981 census data, and rates are given per 1000 population.

of met demand; as an average, it was observed to vary by a factor of 2–3 between local services. However, average bed use can only reflect the demand on the beds which are provided, not on what is needed. A third aspect – uptake of facilities provided – was not considered, but perhaps should have been, because of concern that more beds may be used simply because more are available, even if they are not strictly needed; such a situation would suggest low cost-effectiveness. Equally, there may be a need for in-patient provision that is not currently being met. Therefore, the level of present bed use clearly cannot be taken as an accurate indication of what is needed and desirable.

Ideally, by looking at the provision of beds in different catchment areas, one might identify the extent to which variation in psychiatric morbidity on the one hand, and underprovision of necessary services on the other, explain variations in bed use. However, the ability to measure psychiatric morbidity, as opposed to admission or contact rates, is limited. Often, bed provision is determined by extraneous forces e.g. the availability of nursing staff, and these become the limiting factors which primarily determine both the pattern of service and its quality.

The first report also identified a number of the factors that were likely to affect bed use: (a) *inflow factors*, such as day hospitals or community nursing services, could reduce the need for admission, but admission of psycho-geriatric and long-stay patients to acute-case wards could misleadingly increase actual bed use; (b) *length-of-treatment factors* reflecting special interests such as in-patient psychotherapy, brief hospital stays, or admission of forensic psychiatry patients; (c) *outflow factors*, which reduce length of stay by allowing for the early transfer of patients to chronic-case units, facilities for homeless persons, etc; and allow for easy discharge, but may create the misleading impression that a unit survives on a low number of acute-case beds, because it is not recognised that patients are simply being transferred to other hospitals or facilities.

The disproportionate effect that longer-stay patients have on bed use was illustrated by the finding (Hirsch, 1983) that if all patients under 65 years of age who stayed in hospital from 6 to 12 months were discharged by 6 months, there would be a 16% saving in acute-case bed use, yet only 5% of admissions need be affected. However, if all admissions staying less than 1 week were not admitted to hospital, bed occupancy would be reduced by only 2%, despite a 20% reduction in admissions.

To get a more accurate assessment of the number of patients who occupy acute-case beds, and of the extent to which the presence or absence of elements of a comprehensive service accounted for differences in bed use, when comparing one service with another, the following studies were carried out:

1. a review of the literature on social indices of psychiatric morbidity in relation to bed usage;
2. a comparison of data from the eight psychiatric case registers, supplied and analysed by the Psychiatric Case Registers Group;
3. a study of 20 DGH-based units, chosen because of the variation in length of stay, to examine in detail what factors account for differences between hospitals in bed use and length of stay.

It was hoped that more detailed and accurate knowledge of services at the extremes of high and low bed provision would enable the working party to determine several factors that need to be taken into account when planning for the size of in-patient units. The other important factor was the level of local psychiatric morbidity, which determines potential need by patients for the service. The actual current use of the service was one indication of bed needs, and this is discussed later. However, given the filter effect described by Goldberg & Huxley (1980), which can itself be affected by local conditions and can distort apparent demands, an independent, readily accessible means of estimating the potential psychiatric demand would be useful.

2 Review of literature on social indicators of psychiatry morbidity and uptake of psychiatric services

Although there was little evidence until recently to confirm a relationship between the socio-demographic characteristics of a population and the population's use of psychiatric services, the relationship between social-class factors and physical disease suggests that the same link should also apply to social-class factors and psychiatry. Medical services in general are more concentrated in larger conurbations, and the demand for psychiatric services is much less in suburbs and rural areas (Paykel, 1978). If this reflects need rather than provision, it would be *prima facie* evidence that the supply of psychiatric services and number of beds should be varied according to the socio-demographic characteristics of the population. However, the problem is that bed use may be affected by a number of other factors that are independent of need, such as hospital admission policies, the desirability of the facility provided, stigma associated with treatment, and the availability of other services that provide alternatives to in-patient treatment.

The relationship of socio-economic variables to the prevalence of psychiatric morbidity

This review relates socio-demographic factors to psychiatric morbidity and the uptake of psychiatric services. It will be apparent that social indices should be taken into account in planning the provision of psychiatric beds.

A considerable literature exists relating to the incidence and prevalence of specific psychiatric conditions in different population groups. For example, Faris & Dunham (1939) found that admission rates for schizophrenia were higher in city centres than the suburbs, while affective disorders have been shown to have a higher-than-average incidence in seamen and in male university students (Bagley, 1973). There is evidence that alcoholism has a higher incidence in the lowest social class – after adjusting for other factors (Goodman *et al* 1983). Migration is among the contributory factors to higher prevalence rates (Odegard, 1932; Cochrane, 1977), because under certain circumstances those with greatest risk have a greater tendency to migrate, and because those who migrate may come to live in more provocative circumstances. Dunham (1965) has shown that patients with schizophrenia are more geographically mobile, possibly because of a tendency to separate from cultural roots. Others have shown the importance of social drift, which is a tendency of those affected by mental disorder to drift down the socio-economic scale, and to end up living under more deprived social conditions than those from which they originated (Goldberg & Morrison, 1963). However, in the case of alcoholism, there appears to be a greater aetiological risk in those with low socio-economic status (Goodman *et al*, 1983), even after social drift has been taken into account.

A relationship between ethnic groups and migration has also been observed in parasuicide. In a retrospective study of 4770 admissions for parasuicide in Birmingham over a 4-year period (Burke, 1976), citizens of the Irish Republic and Northern Ireland had a much higher rate than West Indians and Asians, who had the same rate as other UK citizens. However, the parasuicide rates for all three ethnic groups were higher than those reported in these ethnic groups in their indigenous environment. Thus, migration seems to have led here to an increased rate of parasuicide, but there are differences between ethnic groups in their susceptibility, so that the overall National Census category percentage of 'non-UK born' may not necessarily be a useful indicator of psychiatric morbidity.

The observation that social indicators are correlated with variations in admission or in morbidity figures suggests the possibility that social factors can be identified that relate to an increased prevalence of psychiatric disorder, and that planners will need to take this into account. If that is the case, then the presence or absence of these factors should help planners to opt for a corresponding psychiatric bed provision for the population in their area. However, although the evidence demonstrating higher rates of schizophrenia in migrants, and in people living in poorer areas of conurbations, is relevant to estimating the size of resources needed, it is a step away from the problem of estimating the overall need for more facilities; this is because it deals only with increased rates for certain diagnostic groups.

Unemployment is another factor which may affect morbidity. In a study by the Medical Research Council/Social Science Research Council (MRC/SSRC) Social and Applied Psychology Unit in Sheffield, the mental-health status of a sample of school-leavers was assessed before they left school, and again after they had been in the labour market for 12–18 months (Nuffield/York Portfolio Series, 1985). It was found that those who were still unemployed after 18 months had worse mental health than those who were not. Evidence from this study of the effect of mental health on admission rates will be considered later. Further evidence of the effect of unemployment on psychiatric morbidity comes from a recent study by Platt & Kreitman (1985), which showed a positive and highly significant association between unemployment and parasuicide rates, persisting over time and across geographical areas. The highest relative risk was found among the long-term unemployed, but there was a marked increase in parasuicide rates among those who had recently lost their jobs, compared with the employed. The parasuicide rate among the unemployed was nearly always more than ten times higher than that for the employed.

Dohrenwend & Dohrenwend (1975), in a study of mental illness in New York City, observed that the highest overall rates for psychiatric disorders were found in the lowest socio-economic class, and this observation finds support in the UK.

Buglass *et al* (1980) examined a wide range of variables relating to hospital in-patient admissions: these included social problems, data from the former Public Health Department, education, the rateable value of domestic properties, rates of suicidal behaviour, notifications to the Children's Reporter, eviction orders, electricity disconnections, and a selection of 1971 National Census data for the City of Edinburgh. The data were analysed by municipal wards: the three highest 'problem scores' occurred in three wards which were more disadvantaged than the other areas of the city, while parasuicide correlated negatively with two items – rateable value of domestic property, and the number of owner-occupier households. In effect, areas where property was of a higher rateable value, and where there were a large number of owner-occupiers, showed a lower parasuicide rate.

Social indicators of service use and need

So far, social indicators have been considered in relation to rates for a particular illness, or for the severity of illness. Evidence will not be examined which directly relates social indicators to the uptake of psychiatric services.

Hassall (pers. comm.) examined admission rates from both urban and rural areas in Worcestershire, and found marked differences in the admission rates from the two types of environment. For the under 65s, the admission rates from rural areas range from 215 per 100 000 to just over 300 per 100 000; while for the urban group, admission rates range from 332 per 100 000 to 444 per 100 000. Similar differences emerged for the over-65 group, the admission rate from rural areas ranging from 360 per 100 000 to 640 per 100 000, while the rates from urban areas ranged from 530 per 100 000 to 1060 per 100 000. These rates were recorded over a 7-year period from 1976 to 1982 (see Table II).

Buglass *et al* (1980) found a correlation between groups of National Census variables and sub-group scores relating to specific problem areas. The former combined various items from the 1971 Census data to form three principal census components: one reflected isolation and poor social integration; a second related to deprivation; and a third was to do with the age–sex status of the population. The sub-group scores comprised eight separate clusters of variables, in which all those within one sub-group appeared to relate to each other and to be derived from specific problem areas, such as handicap, poverty, and mental-hospital experience; this latter sub-group was derived mainly from data on hospital admission rates

TABLE II
Worcester Development Project: Admission rates per 100 000 population (1976–1982)

	Urban		Rural	
	< 65 years	*65 years and over*	*< 65 years*	*65 years and over*
1976	344.6	543.7	239.4	359.6
1977	332.6	529.8	224.7	463.2
1978	367.7	853.6	236.1	488.5
1979	406.6	886.1	230.4	641.6
1980	444.2	842.8	302.7	584.5
1981	332.0	1066.0	248.3	527.2
1982	418.5	1059.0	214.8	527.2

for a range of psychiatric disorders. The authors noted a reasonably high positive correlation between the mental-hospital scores and both the first two census components, i.e. social isolation and deprivation. However, in the rank order for the mental-hospital sub-group, a relatively advantaged ward, which came fairly low down in the rank order for such items as poverty and problems relating to children and adolescents, nevertheless came relatively high (6 out of 23) on the 'mental hospital' score. A possible reason for this was that the main psychiatric hospital for the city was situated in a particular ward. In other words, proximity to psychiatric facilities may play a part in the extent to which they are used.

The report by Gibbons *et al* (1983) states that in local planning, three interacting groups of factors must be taken into account. These are: changes in the size, composition, and age-structure of the population; special aspects of the development of local services; and (of relevance here), socio-demographic characteristics of the population – such as indices of poverty, social isolation, rural *vs* urban location, and ethnicity. The report examines a number of social indices taken from the 1981 Census indicators, including social isolation, single-parent families, overcrowding, status as an owner-occupier as opposed to council or other tenant, and lack of an exclusive bath/WC, etc. It suggests that the seven English and Welsh Register areas could be divided into three groups: the decaying inner-city areas, such as Camberwell and Salford; industrial/commercial cities, such as Southampton, Nottingham, and Cardiff; prosperous areas of population growth, such as Worcester and Oxford. The latter stood out as being relatively privileged on several indicators, e.g. housing conditions and fewer single parents, while Camberwell stood out as markedly less privileged on almost every indicator.

If indices of psychiatric-bed use are examined, a number of features emerge. The Worcester area consistently showed the lowest in-patient admission rate per 100 000 population throughout the 6 years under study; Camberwell had the second highest rate; and the highest was in Southampton. However, these rates are for the total population aged 15 and over. When the population is broken down to show age-specific rates for those aged 15–64 and those aged 65 and over, Camberwell emerges as having the highest admission rate for adults aged 15–64, while Southampton has a consistently very high rate for those aged 65 and over. Similarly, Camberwell had the highest rates per 100 000 population for short-stay resident in-patients aged between 15 and 64, while Worcester had the lowest rates. This also applied to the medium long-stay group aged 15–64, i.e. patients in hospital between 1 and 5 years.

In 1983, the Nottinghamshire County Council published a study which divided Nottingham into zones of approximately 3000 population, and examined a number of indicators of disadvantage for each zone (S. Jones, I. L. Kontny & J. Cooper, pers. comm.). These indicators included indices of low income, unemployment, lack of skills, poor housing, poor health, and family problems. When the zones were grouped into social-service areas, and the psychiatric-service utilisation from each social-service area was studied, a strong correlation was found between indicators of disadvantage and service-utilisation rates. Almost 80% of the county zones in the social-service areas with the highest utilisation rates were defined as 'disadvantaged', 76% being of extreme or serious disadvantage. In contrast, there were no zones of extreme or serious disadvantage in the areas with the lowest use of service, and only one of moderate disadvantage.

The Nuffield/York Portfolio Series report (1985) suggests that there may be some correlation between the uptake of mental-health services and unemployment.

This extends the observations of a relationship between social indices and parasuicide rates to the expected consequence – an increase in contact with, and admission to, psychiatric facilities. It is not suggested that there is any direct correlation between measures of mental health in the population and levels of unemployment, but there appears to be some correlation between unemployment and admissions to mental-health facilities. Thus it would appear that increases in admissions following unemployment do not necessarily reflect worsening mental health; they may, for example, reflect a greater opportunity to seek treatment. Alternatively, it is suggested that unemployment may make it less easy for others to tolerate or support an individual's symptoms, and lead to pressure on them to seek treatment.

Kangesu *et al* (pers. comm.) carried out a study of 74 patients admitted to Springfield Hospital, South London, over a 9-month period from four electoral wards (two from well-off areas where less than 9% of the population live in council houses and less than 4% are unemployed, and two from areas where 57% and 82% live in council houses and 13–14% are unemployed). Age-related expected admission rates were calculated for each ward: the two more-deprived wards had a 59% and 72% increase in observed admissions, compared with expected rates. There was an increase in both new- and established-case admissions from the less-affluent areas, but more so due to established cases. This might be predicted if social factors

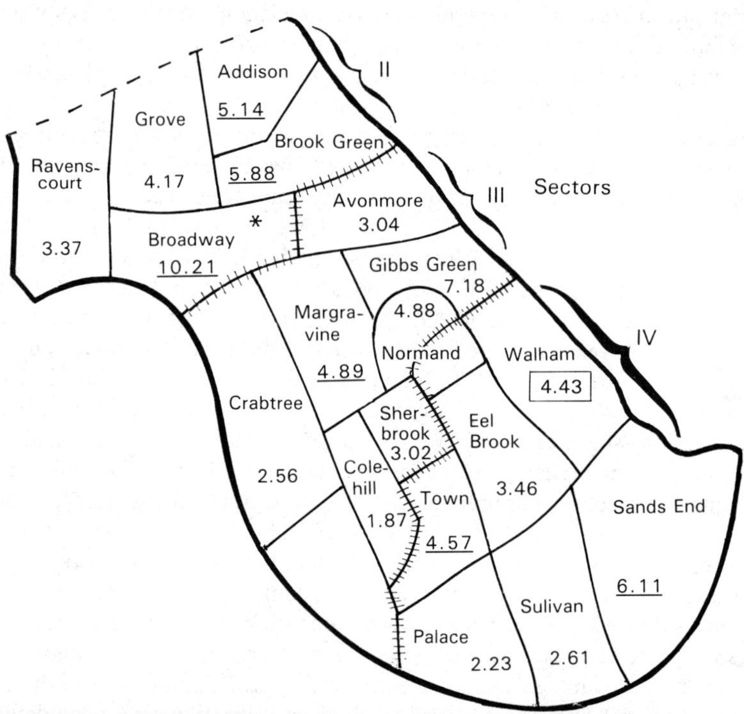

*Fig. 1 South Hammersmith Health District's admission rates per 1000 population for each ward. The mean admission rate was 4.42, boxed in the figure where it occurs. Rates above the mean are underlined. Consultant sectors are divided from each other by '''' marks. ——— , borough boundary; ———, ward boundary. The distribution of admission rates shows that the sectors are evenly distributed for high and low admission rates, so the consultant and clinical team responsible for a sector do not account for the high or low discharge rate. *, Charing Cross Hospital.*

increase the extent of mental illness in certain areas, and are related to increased rates of relapse and lower support and provision outside hospital. Admission to private hospitals and cross-boundary flows were not corrected for, but the magnitude of the differences was so great – six times as many patients were admitted from the more-deprived areas – that it is unlikely that as many patients as this were admitted to alternative facilities.

One of the criticisms of using admission figures as an indicator of morbidity is that the available resources of the service, and admission policies, affect admission rates. The above study partly overcomes that problem, because it looks at differences between sectors having different social profiles admitted to the same hospital with approximately the same resources, social-work support, and local authorities. Although consultants for the different sectors may have had somewhat differing policies, these differences were probably marginal, so that the study gives evidence of a higher admission rate from more socially deprived areas.

A more detailed study, again confirming the close relationship between social deprivation and admission rates, was recently carried out by Foster (pers. comm.) for the Hammersmith & Fulham Health District. The analysis by electoral ward of all admissions from South Hammersmith in 1984 revealed a nearly six-fold variation in admissions per 1000 population – from 1.87 to 10.21. These differences were not explicable by a difference in clinical policies, since the variations applied within the clinical sectors (see Fig. 1), the same resources were used by all clinical teams, and they were served by the same local-authority resources. Table III shows that admissions from each ward were about equally distributed to acute-case beds, which went on a first-come-first-served basis to Charing Cross Hospital, with the 'overflow' going to Banstead Hospital in Surrey. Admission rates were highly

TABLE III

Psychiatric admissions to Charing Cross and Banstead Hospitals (1984): by electoral ward in South Hammersmith

Electoral ward	Charing Cross	Banstead	Total	Admissions per 1000 population	Rank	Jarman score	Jarman rank
Ravenscourt	11	7	18	3.37	12	20.48	12
Grove	15	10	25	4.17	10	29.78	7
Addison	21	15	36	5.48	5	33.31	3
Brook Green	22	13	35	5.88	4	26.82	10
Broadway	25	22	47	10.21	1	34.02	2
Avonmore	14	4	18	3.04	13	29.57	8
Crabtree	7	6	13	2.56	16	12.06	18
Margravine	17	6	23	4.84	7	32.34	5
Gibbs Green	26	20	46	7.18	2	30.67	6
Normand	19	11	30	4.88	6	39.88	1
Palace	7	5	12	2.23	17	13.11	17
Colehill	6	5	11	1.87	18	17.97	15
Sherbrooke	11	4	15	3.02	14	17.71	16
Walham	12	16	28	4.43	9	26.08	11
Town	15	12	27	4.57	8	18.55	13
Eel Brook	14	7	21	3.46	11	27.26	9
Sulivan	8	7	15	2.61	15	18.31	14
Sands End	22	11	33	6.11	3	32.99	4
South Hammersmith sub-total	272	181	453	4.42			

TABLE IV
20-Hospitals' study: ranking of service indicators

(A) Hospitals (ranked by number of beds)	(B) Discharges per 1000 population ranked	(C) Rankings of numbers of beds	(D) Rankings of activity	(E) Rankings of resources	(F) Jarman UPA score ranked	(G) Jarman UPA scores
1	4	1	1	1	3	17.60
2	3	2	4	2	1	48.62
3	2	3	3	4	15	−7.62
4	16	4	14	5	19	−26.59
5	14	5	12	5	18	−20.55
6	1	6	2	7	6	13.86
7	11	7	14	3	20	−32.79
8	13	8	8	7	9	3.80
9	8	9	6	9	8	8.21
10	6	10	8	13	10	−1.99
11	5	11	4	10	4	17.25
12	18	12	16	12	7	10.83
13	10	13	6	18	2	35.75
14	9	14	10	17	13	−5.71
15	7	15	12	15	11	−3.00
16	20	16	20	11	12	−5.54
17	12	17	10	16	14	−6.15
18	17	18	19	20	5	15.94
19	15	19	16	14	17	−12.32
20	19	20	16	19	16	−9.08

The Districts are ranked by their Jarman score (column F)
They are compared with the ranking on discharge per 1000 population (column B)

correlated ($r=0.82$) with social deprivation factors, as represented by the Underprivileged Area (UPA) score devised by Jarman (1983, 1984). This comprises a weighted composite of eight census variables of social deprivation: elderly living alone; under 5s; one-parent families, unskilled workers; unemployed people; overcrowded homes; people recently having moved house; ethnic minorities. The same exercise has been carried out as part of the comparison of 20 DGH-based hospitals studied for this report. The correlation between discharge rate and Jarman UPA score was $r=0.41$. The correlation was at a lower but significant ($P=0.05$) level, even though the areas differed in level of resources and type of service. Also, there was no correction for cross-boundary flow, and the district UPA scores used did not always correspond to the psychiatric catchment areas (see Table IV). Mental Health Enquiry data were used to perform an analysis of all adult psychiatric admissions in 1984 from the North West Thames Regional Health Authority; the data were tabulated by district-of-residence, and therefore were not affected by cross-boundary flow. The districts of the region span almost the entire range of Jarman UPA scores. Total adult district admission rates and district admission rates for the under-65s correlated with Jarman UPA scores ($r=0.76$ and $r=0.8$, respectively) (see Table V). There is therefore a strong relationship between psychiatric admission rates and indices of social deprivation.

Discussion and summary

The studies reviewed here suggest a strong association between the uptake of psychiatric services and a variety of socio-demographic factors, including: residence

TABLE V
The North West Thames Regional Health Authority's 1984 district admission rates and UPA scores

District health authority	'UPA 8VARS'	Rank of 'UPA 8VARS'	Adult admission per 1000 population	Rank adult admission rate	Adult admission under 65 years per 1000 population	Rank adult admission under 65 years
Paddington & N. Kensington	44.80	1	5.61	2	4.90	2
Hammersmith & Fulham	31.76	2	5.58	3	4.86	3
Brent	18.67	3	3.72	8	3.03	6
Victoria	18.57	4	6.97	1	5.58	1
Ealing	14.77	5	4.21	5	3.32	5
South Beds	−2.02	6	3.85	6	2.59	7
Hounslow & Spelthorne	−3.47	7	3.17	10	2.49	8
Barnet	−6.97	8	3.21	9	2.37	10
North Beds	−8.16	9	3.15	10	2.11	12
Hillingdon	−9.05	10	2.98	12	2.26	11
North Herts	−11.74	11	3.73	7	2.42	9
Harrow	−13.17	12	4.73	4	3.38	4
SW Herts	−19.26	13	2.62	14	1.49	15
NW Herts	−20.69	14	2.83	13	1.85	13
East Herts	−26.59	15	2.55	15	1.81	14

Spearman rank order correlation coefficients: total adult admissions with 'UPA 8VARS' (people from underprivileged area – eight variables), $r=0.76$; adult admissions under 65 years with UPA 8VARS $r=0.8$

in city centres; lower social class; social deprivation; social isolation; the proportion of immigrant families; single-parent families; overcrowding; low income; percentage of owner-occupier housing; poor housing; council housing; and (of particular importance in recent years) high rates of unemployment. The social mobility of the population, which can be measured in terms of the percentage of the population who change residence very 3 years, is a useful indicator of the 'conurbation factor', whereby people with increased risk and less social support tend to concentrate themselves in certain areas of large cities. This increases the pressure on admission services, particularly for alcoholism and schizophrenia, and shows as an increased length of stay, since this group is more difficult to discharge quickly back to the community.

Thus, if the correlations observed between admission rates and social-deprivation scores in Hammersmith and North West Thames Regional Health Authority, using Jarman's method, were replicated in other regions, this might become a powerful tool for estimating the potential psychiatric demand for services in every district. Jarman is able to provide scores of social deprivation (UPA score) for all catchment areas and 192 health districts in the UK, as the method depends on available census data for 9265 electoral wards; a district need only compare its score with the national distribution of Jarman scores in other districts. Appendix 1 includes a table of UPA scores for all districts in the UK. The corresponding discharge rates given in Table XXII may serve as a guide to other districts.

It does not necessarily follow for every area that high social deprivation, even if associated with an increased prevalence or severity of mental illness, leads to increased demand for services. This is illustrated by the link between rates for schizophrenia and migration. The presence of immigrant communities may be associated with increased admission rates from some groups, but not others, as found by Burke (1976). However, other immigrant groups may have lower admission rates, because they provide a more stable environment for individuals within their own communities, or because they are pre-selected for lower risk when they migrate, or because their cultural values discourage use of local psychiatric services, or a combination of these factors.

Other factors, such as the proximity and accessibility of the service, may increase or decrease demand, and may in some instances be more important than, for example, socio-economic factors. Thus, Buglass *et al* (1980) found a high admission rate from populations which were close to a psychiatric teaching hospital, although this population was relatively low on indices of poverty and problems relating to children and adolescents. This points to the need for a local adjustment of predicted demand, based on a knowledge of local circumstances.

It is the prevalence, rather than the incidence, of psychiatric morbidity that planners need to know in order to plan services; many of the difficult issues of cause and effect that are important to epidemiologists interested in social causes of mental illness are therefore not directly of concern. Thus, it is possible that worse social conditions might increase the demand for admission (or slow the rate of discharge) without causing increased rates of psychiatric morbidity, while an investment in improving social conditions might increase demand. The specific concern here is about demand, whatever the cause, and the recognition that a variety of responses is possible.

The most relevant findings in this review all show a several-fold difference in admission rates in small populations with high and low indices, of socio-economic deprivation – a factor which is often obscured by using larger population groupings based on census figures. Clearly, there are advantages in having accurate population data for small population units, with corresponding hospital admission rates and other data for the same populations, and Jarman's work (1983, 1984) seems to have made this possible.

While use reflects demand to a greater or lesser extent, it cannot necessarily be taken to reflect need. This raises conceptual issues as to how to define 'need'. There are clear distinctions between: areas where there is little demand because the service is lacking or unacceptable; areas where the service is accessible and able to meet demand; areas where the population tends not to use the service, despite adequate provision; and, perhaps, areas that are overprovided for, in the sense that facilities are used in a way that is not cost-effective because of inefficient practice.

3 The case-register study

Case registers are based on catchment-area populations, and describe the total care each patient receives, wherever treated. They thereby overcome the problem of cross-boundary flows and distortions that might occur because part of the catchment-area population receives treatment at other hospitals or because a catchment area receives patients from other districts. At the time of this study, there were eight psychiatric case registers in the UK, five of which served populations with a DGH. Such a register provides the best available data on the resources used by a defined population. This can be compared with the results of the working party's survey of 20 hospitals, which depended on less-precise data-gathering techniques, based on the services provided by a district (for the purpose of this report, catchment-area services and district services will be used synonymously to refer to the totality of National Health Service provision for a specified local population). The data were supplied with the approval of the case-register directors, and the analysis was carried out by Mr C. Jennings. Each case register was separately analysed for all discharges in 1981, allowing for comparison with the working party's retrospective analysis of 400 discharged patients in 1981 from each of the 20 hospitals visited.

Resident in-patients per 1000 population

Table VI (columns D and E) shows the number of patients from each register's catchment area occupying a psychiatric bed anywhere on 31 December 1981, per 1000 population of the register area. Because of the census day chosen, this may represent a slight underestimate of beds usually in use. For the age-group 15–64, the mean is 0.39 beds per 1000 population, with a range of usage from 0.19 per 1000 beds in Worcester to 0.76 per 1000 beds in Camberwell. The proportion of patients treated in a DGH unit within a catchment area is shown in Table VI. Table VI also shows that, on average across the register areas, nearly 34% of all adult psychiatric beds for patients staying up to 1 year are used by the elderly, aged over 65. Thus, any service which does not have adequate provision for this group will be putting a severe burden on the rest of the acute psychiatric service. Finally, Table VI shows the number of patients discharged from DGHs as a percentage of total discharges from the catchment area (column C).

TABLE VI
Psychiatric case-register data (1981)

	(A)	(B)	(C)	(D)	(E)
				Total bed occupancy <1 year anywhere per 1000 population	
	DGH	Total	Percentage DGH	Age 15–64	Age 15 and over
Worcester	1057	1076	98	0.19	0.42
Oxford	162	2256	7	0.21	0.37
Salford	321	898	36	0.34	0.70
Southampton	795	1411	56	0.36	0.70
Cardiff	195	1021	19	0.38	0.65
Nottingham	—	1543	0	0.38	0.70
Aberdeen	—	2766	0	0.50	1.02
Camberwell	—	644	0	0.76	1.27
Mean ±s.d.				0.39±0.18	0.73±0.29

NB DGH discharges include tranfers to local hospitals, other than the DGH, whereas the count of total discharges ignores such transfers. Thus, the DGH count is not strictly a subset of the total count, and the percentages are slightly inflated. The average number of beds per 1000 population occuped by people aged 65 and over is $(0.73-0.39)=0.34$. To estimate the average number of beds available, the figures need to be increased by approximately 15% to allow for 85% occupancy, i.e. 0.46 per 1000 for age 15–64 and 0.86 per 1000 for 15 and over.

TABLE VII
Percentage of in-patients discharged within or staying longer than a specified period (1981): Psychiatric case register data (1981)

	<1 week		<12 weeks		>24 weeks		>1 year	
	Total	DGH	Total	DGH	Total	DGH	Total	DGH
Worcester	16	17	90	92	6	5	4	2.5
Oxford	38	35	90	97	6	1	3	0
Salford	18	22	88	99	7	0	4	0
Southampton	24	40	92	94	5	3	3	0.3
Cardiff	23	29	85	93	11	2	8	1.0
Nottingham	15	—	83	—	9	—	6	—
Aberdeen	17	—	—	—	12(>26 weeks)		8	—
Camberwell	12	—	73	—	14	—	6	—

Total refers to the percentage discharged from all hospitals; *DGH* refers to the percentage discharged from DGH units serving the register population.

Worcester and Oxford have the lowest bed use of the register areas, but Worcester depends on the DGH for 98% of beds and Oxford for only 7%. It follows that the presence of a DGH-based unit, in itself, does not explain the variation in bed use.

Table VII shows the percentage of patients discharged within various periods of time after admission, comparing the percentage discharged from the DGH with the percentage discharged from all beds serving the district. A higher proportion of DGH-treated patients are discharged sooner than mental-hospital-based patients, regardless of the register area. However, these differences are slight, and might be due to differences in the type and severity of cases differentially admitted to the DGH as compared with the mental hospital, when both are available. These figures are generally higher than the figures from the 20-hospital study.

TABLE VIII

Resident in-patients (1981) per 1000 population by length of stay: Psychiatric case register data (1981)

	Length of stay		
	< 2 months	*< 1 year*	*1–5 years*
Age 15 and over			
Camberwell	0.53	1.27	0.56
Salford	0.30	0.70	0.58
Southampton	0.46	0.70	0.37
Nottingham	0.37	0.70	0.37
Cardiff	0.39	0.65	0.48
Worcester	0.25	0.42	0.20
Oxford	0.18	0.37	0.18
Aberdeen	0.48	1.02	0.71
Mean ±s.d.		0.73±0.29	0.43±0.18
England	—	0.57	0.37
Wales	—	0.57	0.34
Scotland	—	0.87	0.82
Age 15–64			
Camberwell	0.41	0.76	0.20
Salford	0.19	0.34	0.18
Southampton	0.23	0.36	0.17
Nottingham	0.21	0.38	0.14
Cardiff	0.25	0.38	0.14
Worcester	0.13	0.19	0.05
Oxford	0.11	0.21	0.06
Aberdeen	0.26	0.50	0.24
Mean ±s.d.		0.39±0.18	0.15±0.07
England	—	0.31	0.13
Wales	—	0.31	0.12
Scotland	—	0.46	0.26

TABLE IX

Percentage of diagnostic group among in-patient discharges (1981) by diagnosis and age (15–64): Psychiatric case register data (1981)

	Schizophrenia	Affective disorders	Alcohol and drug problems	Neurosis (not depression)	Personality disorders	Other
Worcester	20	42	15	3	7	11
Oxford	13	22	44	5	10	6
Salford	24	41	9	11	12	5
Southampton	19	42	16	6	8	10
Cardiff	23	32	14	9	7	16
Nottingham	22	42	16	5	6	9
Aberdeen	16	32	24	4	14	10
Camberwell	24	40	10	5	5	16

Table VIII shows the bed occupancy for in-patients aged 15 and over, and aged 15–64, within specified periods of length of stay. The register areas have, on average, higher bed use than England and Wales, but not Scotland.

Diagnosis

Table IX shows the diagnostic distribution for the 15–64 age-group. There is no relationship between the percentage of patients in different diagnostic groups

TABLE X

Clinical activity: bed use vs discharges: out-patients seen; domiciliary visits; rates per 1000 total population; Psychiatric case register data (1981)

	Resident in-patients		Discharges	NHS day-care patients at 31 December 1981	Out-patients seen per 1000 population	Domiciliary visits per 1000 population	Community psychiatric nurse contacts per 1000 population
	<1 year	<5 year					
Worcester	0.42	0.62	3.3	0.47	6.04	1.99	3.19
Oxford	0.37	0.55	4.5	0.95	—	0.69	—
Salford	0.70	1.28	3.7	0.59	10.1	1.68	6.11
Southampton	0.70	1.07	6.9	0.67	8.13	5.63	3.55
Cardiff	0.65	1.13	3.7	—	5.93	—	—
Nottingham	0.70	1.07	4.1	0.76	9.09	1.41	1.64
Aberdeen	1.02	1.73	5.2	—	—	—	—
Camberwell	1.27	1.83	5.1	0.63	—	—	—
Mean ±s.d.	0.73±0.29	1.16±0.46	4.56±1.2				

within each register area, and the ranking of the area on bed/population ratios. This is also true for the over-65 age-group. For example, Worcester and Salford, with the lowest and third-lowest bed occupancy, respectively, have a high percentage of patients with schizophrenia, while Oxford (second lowest) has a low percentage of patients with psychosis and a high percentage of patients with alcoholism.

Clinical activity

Table X shows the total bed-occupancy-per-1000-population ratios for patients over 15 years, those resident less than 1 year, and those for less than 5 years, including ESMI patients, and their relationship to other indicators of clinical activity. This table incorporates data from Tables VI and VII. Although the *acute*-case-beds-per-1000-population ratio for patients staying less than 1 year is strongly correlated with the bed ratio for *all patients*, including ESMI (correlation between resident in-patients < 1 and < 5 years is $r = 0.77$), there are no consistent relationships between bed-occupancy ratios and the other indicators of clinical activity shown. The correlation of acute-case bed ratios with overall discharge rates is low ($r = 0.39$ for all patients, and 0.36 for ages 15–64). For patients staying up to 1 year, $r = 0.26$. Notwithstanding this apparently low correlation, certain extreme values suggest a possible contribution of discharge rates to low or high bed ratios.

Worcester, with the lowest bed ratio, has a much lower proportion of day patients, and a relatively low number of domiciliary visits, out-patients, and community psychiatric-nurse visits, relative to Salford and Southampton. This suggests a relatively low overall level of clinical activity; however, Nottingham, which has a relatively high bed use, has a high proportion of day patients, and the second highest out-patient-clinic activity. Southampton has a generally high discharge rate and high levels of activity, suggesting it is a 'high-efficiency' clinical service, in the sense of showing high levels of activity but only moderate use of hospital beds. There does not seem to be any simple, direct relationship between use of beds and any single service variable shown in Table XI, given the number of day patients, out-patients, domiciliary visits, or community psychiatric-nurse contacts – each shown as a ratio per 1000 population. Further data, not shown here, indicate that the proportion of patients admitted under the Mental Health Act has no bearing on the differences in bed occupancy of the case-register areas – the percentages detained are low, with little variation among the eight register areas.

TABLE XI
Mental-illness hospitals and units in England (1982)

Age group	Acute cases	New long-stay	Established long-stay	Total
Occupied beds				
0–64	15 245	10 846	8111	34 202
65 and over	12 370	15 344	11 298	39 012
All ages	27 615	26 190	19 409	73 214
Rates per 100 000 population				
0–64	38	27	20	86
65 and over	174	216	159	549
All ages	59	56	41	156

The above estimates are based on an updating of the 1971 *Mental Health Enquiry* census; they are therefore not precise figures, and should be regarded as doing little more than indicating the order of magnitude involved

Conclusion from survey of case-register population

Case registers provide the most accurate way of estimating the uptake of psychiatric services by a target population, because they account for the total use of services by their population, both within and outside the catchment area; therefore, they overcome the problems created by cross-boundary flow. While the case-register districts were not representative for the UK as a whole, they included diversified service styles, as well as urban and rural locations, and varied according to social class and other factors, corresponding to the working party's 20-hospital sample. Indeed, the mean and distribution of bed-per-population ratios is very similar to those of the 20-hospital study, reported below. The mean acute-case bed occupancy for the register sample for patients in hospital under 1 year, age 15–64, is 0.39 ± 0.18 per 1000 population, estimating a bed provision of about 0.46 beds per 1000, after allowing for an occupancy rate of 85%.

The most salient points to emerge from the case-register data regarding factors which may determine bed usage are as follows:

(a) The mean bed occupancy for general psychiatric patients, aged 15–64, for all diagnoses, was 0.39 beds per 1000 population (range 0.19–0.76 per 1000) or 0.73 per 1000 for patients of all ages over 15. This would correspond to an expected bed requirement of 0.46 beds per 1000 population, allowing for 85% occupancy.

(b) Of general psychiatric beds used by patients over 15 years of age, including ESMI, 41% are used by patients aged 65 or more. Any service which does not have adequate facilities for the elderly will put a greater burden on its acute-case general psychiatric beds.

(c) Variations in bed use are not explained by whether the beds are sited in a DGH or mental hospital, although geographical location could be a factor. DGH patients are discharged slightly sooner than mental-hospital-treated patients, regardless of the catchment area, but this may be due to differences in the severity of the disorders for which patients are admitted, when both hospitals are available in the same district.

(d) The proportion of patients from a particular diagnostic group does not explain the variation in bed occupancy, nor does the proportion detained under the Mental Health Act.

(e) Bed occupancy does not correlate well with discharge rates ($r = 0.39$), the number of patients listed as receiving day care or the number per unit of population of out-patient visits, domiciliary visits or community psychiatry nurse visits. However, some relationship between total clinical activity and bed use was evident in particular cases.

(f) In addition, socio-demographic factors and indicators of poverty are correlated with admission rates, which has a bearing on bed use (Gibbons *et al*, 1983).

These findings provide a perspective from which the 20-hospital-study's findings can be compared, and support the conclusions and recommendations in chapters 7 and 8.

4 The twenty-hospital study

The need for an in-depth study of local services

Data that generate information on the number of beds used by different hospitals, districts, and regions are regularly collected by the DHSS. Data such as those in Table I were based on the Mental Health Enquiry, which came from hospital reports of beds in use on 31 December each year. Since no distinction is made for cross-boundary flows, figures from certain districts may be misleadingly high, because they include patients from other districts or regions; correspondingly, those from other districts may be misleadingly low, because a proportion of the patients have been treated in another district's hospitals.

For example, the Camberwell register reported that 30% of patients from its catchment area were treated outside its district, and a similar figure was noted by Hirsch & Kramer in an unpublished survey of patients from an outer-London catchment area. Moreover, the Mental Health Enquiry does not distinguish new long-stay patients and psychogeriatric patients from acutely ill patients, if they are in an acute-case unit. Often, the number of acutely ill patients reported as in-patient is either underreported (because some are boarded-out in non-acute-case wards), or overreported (because patients are on leave but still counted). Where psychogeriatric patients have been in a hospital less than a year, they will be included in the acute-case category, if they are not on a psychogeriatric ward.

Planning can be made more efficient if provision is geared to the needs of specific groups of patients. The original DHSS guideline of 0.5 beds per 1000 population for acute-case beds had not, in recent years, been taken as including the elderly severely mentally infirm (ESMI) who require continuing care, children, adolescents, or the requirements for interim secure units. However, the guideline was meant to include functional patients over 65 years old, and has come to be regarded as excluding provision for patients staying more than 1 or 2 years.

Therefore, there was an obvious need to take a more detailed and consistent look at acute-case bed use, in order to determine the discrepancy between the actual and reported figures for acutely ill patients, as well as to confirm the extent of variation in different localities. At the same time, it was hoped that by simultaneously studying a whole range of factors that might influence demand and use for acute-psychiatric-case beds, more suitable planning and guidance procedures might be devised, including estimates of the effect on bed use where the new pattern of service has been developed.

Hirsch (1983) argued that, in practice, norms are usually based on a 'best estimate'; this takes into account a combination of average current provision that is taken up (current met demand) plus a projection of recent trends, skewed in the direction of current policy. Despite the problems in estimating accurate bed use in different categories from Mental Health Enquiry data at local, district and regional levels, a relevant figure for (national) bed use can readily be obtained within the limits of available census data, as shown in Table XI. However, because these figures are averages, it must be assumed that they represent the mix between hospitals operating traditional services and those operating the new pattern of service (community-orientated psychiatry with less dependence on in-patient care).

One aim of the working party's enquiry was to identify bed needs under conditions of more recent practice in the DGH setting. The 0.5 per 1000 guideline was a forecast: it has proved too high for some new units built to this norm, particularly those outside city centres, and has been all but superseded by a much lower planning figure in the case of some health authorities. It is therefore desirable for those who are planning new units to have knowledge of the range of bed use with the new pattern of service: (a) it is both wasteful to build wards which stand empty, and bad planning if provision is insufficient to meet need; (b) some will argue that the provision of unnecessary beds can create unnecessary demand to keep the beds filled (contrary to the interests of patients), in order to retain resources; (c) an over-estimate of future bed needs increases anticipated building and running costs, as well as adding to the reluctance of the health authorities to allocate finance for the satisfaction of those needs or to give priority to this in their building programmes. If careful study shows that claims to manage satisfactorily with fewer beds are misleading, planners need to know as soon as possible.

The working party decided that it should focus its efforts on determining the planning criteria for acute-case general psychiatric beds for units located within their catchment area. For this reason, it was decided to stratify a sample and to study 20 DGH-based services with high, medium, and low patient turnover rates, in order to maximise differences in bed use.

Aim

The aim of this study was: (a) to identify a suggested *range* of bed provisions for acute cases in adult short-stay general psychiatry, including provision for the elderly with acute functional illnesses, but not for elderly demented patients, long-stay patients (staying more than 1 year), children and adolescents and special units; and (b) to identify factors which will help planners to opt for a high or low figure within the range, according to local circumstances.

Hypotheses

1. There are real differences between psychiatric services in the ratio of beds per population and in throughput, in terms of patients per bed per year; this is after adjusting for beds occupied by patients from outside the catchment area or not used for acute-case general psychiatry (inflow), and adjusting for beds which are in use in other institutions (outflow) and for patients in beds

within units outside the catchment area (cross-boundary flow). The terms
beds per 1000 population, bed-per-population ratio, number of beds, etc. are
used synonymously here.

2. Differences in morbidity (real need) differentiate high from low bed use (inflow
   factors).
3. The availability of ancillary support from local authorities and the voluntary
   sector, in community residential provision, and in alternative services vary
   inversely with bed use (inflow and outflow factors).
4. A community orientation of psychiatric services characterised by more
   community psychiatric nurses, an active domiciliary service, more out-patients,
   walk-in clinics, etc. will be associated with low bed use (outflow and length
   of treatment factors).

Selection of hospitals

From a list including up to three hospitals from each region that had suitable DGH
units with high, medium, and low throughput (patients per year per bed),
respectively, 20 services were selected according to the following criteria: (a) the
units should operate in a DGH and have 50–150 acute-case beds; (b) they should
have about 400 patient-discharges per year or more; (c) the unit should have been
operational for at least 4 years prior to 1981; (d) the unit should have a defined
catchment area and, where possible, should not have a high likelihood of cross-
boundary flow; (e) there should be no known exceptional circumstances operating,
e.g. the unit should not be mainly an early assessment service; (f) some of the units
should demonstrate a high throughput (more than ten patients per bed per year),
some a low throughput (less than six patients per bed per year), and the remainder
should be patients between these limits. Since SH3 (NHS census of bed occupancy)
statistics for 1979 were used to determine the level of throughput, it was not possible
to know whether some ESMI or long-stay patients occupying acute-case beds were
included in the returns (it was, of course, one of the aims of the study to investigate
this); (g) if possible, the units chosen should cover all 14 regions and represent
both urban and rural locations.

The hospitals chosen

Three hospitals had to be withdrawn from the initial short list because they declined
to participate; two others were substituted for them. The final list contained a
few hospitals that did not strictly satisfy the original criteria: according to SH3
statistics, two had 189 and 154 beds, respectively, and a third had only 28 beds.
One hospital had considerable cross-boundary inflow (hospital 1), but this was easy
to take into account.

Table XII shows the original 1979 SH3 data from which the hospitals were chosen
for the study. Table XIII (column B) shows the 1981 figures covering all the
hospitals identified as providing acute-case-bed services to their catchment area. Half
the services had a substantial input of acute-case beds from other sources, which
were not identified when the key hospitals were chosen. Hence, hospital 2A (Table
XII) in the original survey had its beds supplemented by a second hospital, giving
a total of 154 beds, not 80 as was originally believed. The correct numbers of beds
for each catchment area are given in Table XIII, where all acute-case beds in each

TABLE XII

1979 data used to choose the 20 hospitals in the study; as supplied by the DHSS

	Including psychogeriatric beds				Excluding psychogeriatric beds			
(A) Hospital identified by number	*(B)* Beds	*(C)* Patient-discharges per year	*(D)* Patient-discharges per bed	*(E)* Percentage staying over 6 months	*(F)* Beds	*(G)* Patient-discharges per year	*(H)* Percentage occupancy	*(I)* True length of stay in days (adjusted for percentage occupancy)
1A	90	449	5	7	90	449	100	73
2A	80	509	6.4	10	80	509	95	54
3	97	934	9.6	3	97	934	84	32
4	74	467	6.3	3	74	467	66	38
5A	98	604	6.2	—	84	467	73	48
6A	59	802	13.6	1	59	802	76	20
7A	116	761	6.6	—	116	761	77	43
8A	91	504	5.5	4.5	62	334	57	38
9A	55	547	10	9	55	547	84	31
10	60	607	10.1	3	60	607	81	29
11	50	397	7.9	—	50	397	76	35
12A	104	510	4.9	—	89	468	86	60
13A	121	684	5.7	6	121	684	93	60
14A	90	804	8.9	4	90	804	88	36
15	80	1088	13.6	1	80	1088	79	21
16	102	424	4.2	—	102	424	67	59
17	53	436	8.2	—	53	436	72	32
18A	107	561	5.3	6	107	561	89	62
19A	20	309	15.0	—	20	809	67	16
20A	65	676	10.4	5	65	676	74	26

A indicates that the hospital chosen provided only part of the acute-case service

district are combined. Hence hospital 2A in Table XII becomes hospital 2 in Table XIII, while hospital 9A changed from 55 (Table XII) to 78 beds (Table XIII) because Table XII only shows the number of beds in the hospital originally chosen for study.

Survey of 400 consecutive discharges

The hospitals were chosen on the assumption that they provided the acute-case general psychiatry service for their area. However, one aim of the study was to get as accurate a picture as possible of the actual service to the catchment-area population (hereafter referred to as 'the population') and of how the hospital was able to function at either a high or low throughput per bed. The first step, therefore, was to confirm the SH3 data about each hospital, and to determine activity in terms of average length of stay and the contribution of elderly patients to bed-turnover figures.

For this purpose, a survey was carried out which was based on the routine SH3 statistical return for psychiatric in-patients, HMR-1. For each acute-case unit, the last 400 consecutive discharges in 1981 were examined to determine the age, length of stay and other demographic data for each discharge. A pilot exercise at a hospital not included in our survey revealed that, for more than 50% of patients, the diagnostic information relating to outcome was grossly inaccurate, when compared with information based on a direct examination of the clinical case-notes.

Table XIII

Adjustments to determine a standardised number for beds per 1000 population
Psychiatric bed norms

(A) Hospital	(B) 1981 General psychiatric beds SH3	(C) 1981 General psychiatric beds (all)	(D) ESMI assessment and ESMI	(E) Average occupied by new and established long-stay patients	(F) 1981 average acute-case beds	(G) Inflow adjustment excluding non-catchment area	(H) Outflow adjustment, beds in other units	(I) 1981 Census (population in 1000s)	(J) Estimated acute-case beds provided within the district per 1000 population
1	189	160	0	17(5)	143	100	100	177.0	0.56
2	154	118	10*	5	102	93	96	192.4	0.50
3	97	96	0	0	96	86	86	178.0	0.48
4	74	74	12	4	58	43	43	94.1	0.46
5	84	84	0	3	81	80	80	190.5	0.42
6	59	59	(8)	0	50	50	80	188.4	0.42
7	92	72	0	3	69	69	69	166.9	0.41
8	62	54	5	0	54	49	49	120.0	0.41
9	78	78	0	6	72	72	94	234.0	0.40
10	60	60	4*	0	56	56	81	201.0	0.40
11	50	50	4*	4*	46	42	51	130.0	0.39
12	89	88	0	12(3)	76	73	73	189.0	0.39
13	124	79	0	5	74	67	67	179.8	0.37
14	95	95	15(5)	13(2)	77	77	141	468.6	0.30
15	81	79	0	0	79	79	79	288.7	0.27
16	102	96	31	(13)	52	52	54	225.7	0.24
17	53	53	12	0	41	41	41	175.9	0.23
18	107	48	0	0	48	48	63	273.3	0.23
19	28	15	13(3)	0	15	15	24	133.1	0.18
20	83	66	29	4	33	33	33	206.5	0.16
Totals	1761				1323	1192	1371	3806.4	Mean ± s.d. = 0.37 ± 0.08

* No distinction was made between new and established long-stay patients
() Number of established long-stay patients was included in column E and the monitored ESMI assessment beds included in column D are given in parentheses
Column H: outflow adjustment indicates the observed number of acute-case general psychiatry beds (less than 1 year) available for the catchment area on a regular defined basis, excluding ESMI, under 15s and new long-stay patients resident for over 1 year
Inflow: admissions from outside the catchment area; outflow: admissions dealt with outside the catchment area

Results

For the 20 hospitals, there was almost no correlation between the average length of stay (LOS) and the bed provision per 1000 population. The Pearson product–moment correlation was 0.21, which statistically is in the opposite direction to that expected, and is not significant. But it should be no surprise that there is little correlation between throughput-per-bed and bed-to-population ratios, particularly if other hospitals whose beds are not included serve the population, or if acute-case general psychiatry beds have not been distinguished from total 'mental illness' beds. This was the case in several of the services visited.

The concept of throughput – the number of patients per bed in a year – is, by definition, inversely proportional to the average LOS (LOS = 365/patients per bed per year). However, the rank order of hospitals in Tables XIV–XXIII and by LOS in Figs 2–6 does not exactly correspond to the rank order of total acute-case beds in a service per 1000 population, because eight of the twenty districts had their acute-case beds in the key hospital supplemented by beds in other hospitals, which are not taken into account in our study of 400 discharges.

Figure 2 shows the difference between the 20 acute-case units in average LOS of the last 400 discharges in 1981. Average LOS varied from 69 to 16 days per patient (left to right), with a mean LOS of 38 days (s.d. ± 13). Hirsch (1983) found that patients staying more than 6 months make a considerable contribution to the average length of stay of the six hospitals with the longest LOS. For example, hospital A would reduce its length of stay by 30% and hospital C by 40% if all

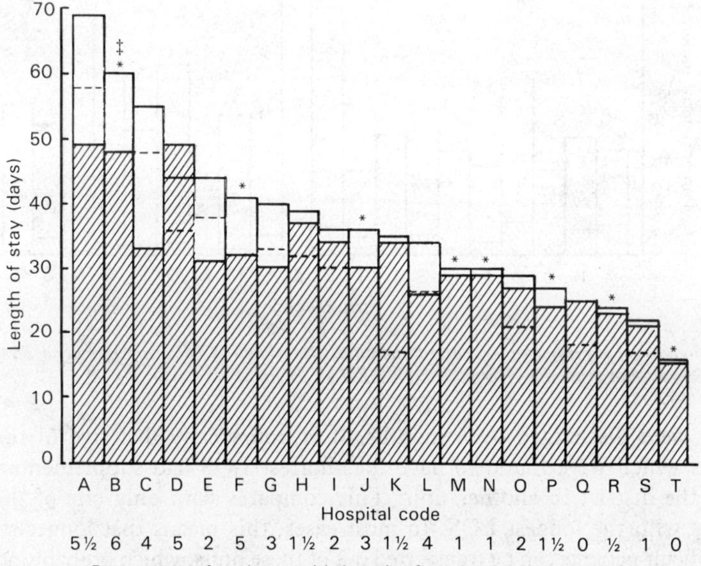

*Fig. 2   Average length of stay of last 400 patients discharged from each of 20 DGH units. The proportion of the average made up by stays over 6 months is shown in white. The order of hospitals A–T does not directly correspond to the ranking of hospitals 1–20 according to the mean number of beds per population in Tables X–XXI. - - -, length of stay after over-65s of all diagnoses are taken out; *, hospitals which either transfer patients out to another facility or have a second acute unit for the population; ‡, two beds for very difficult patients. Key relating hospitals A–T with ranking by bed ratios in Tables X–XXIII; A, 12; B, 16; C, 4; D, 5; E, 1; F, 18; G, 13; H, 7; I, 2; J, 9; K, 8; L, 20; M, 14; N, 10; O, 3; P, 11; Q, 17; R, 19; S, 15; T, 6.*

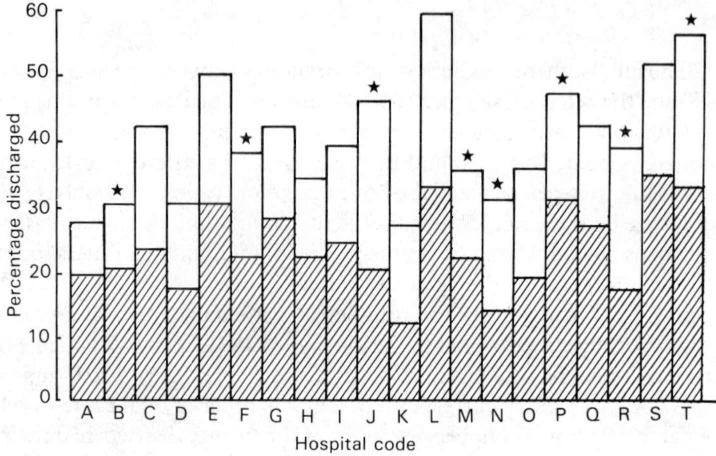

Fig. 3   *Percentage of patients discharged within 2 weeks by hospital.* ▨ *indicates percentage discharged within 1 week. Hospitals are ranked by 'length of stay' (LOS) from highest on the left to lowest on the right, as in Fig. 2. This shows that the proportion of patients discharged within the first 1 or 2 weeks does not determine the differences between hospitals in LOS shown in Fig. 2. ★, indicates hospitals in districts with acute-case beds elsewhere, not accounted for in this Fig.*

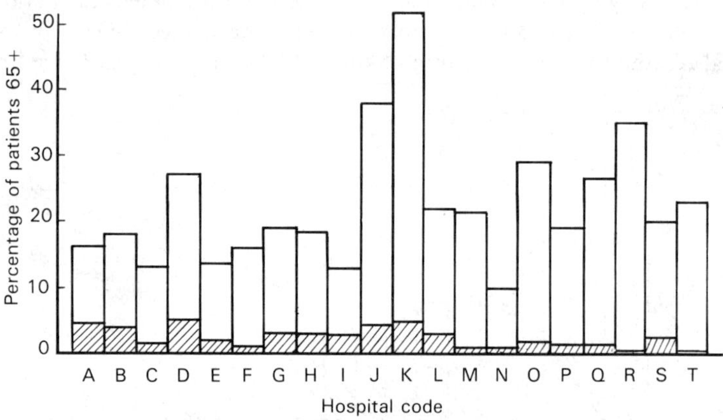

Fig. 4   *Percentage of patients aged 65 or over by hospital. Shaded section indicates percentage of 65 + patients that stay longer than 3 months. Hospitals are ranked by length of stay as in Fig. 2.*

patients were discharged by 6 months. It is noteworthy that five of the eight hospitals which were found to have the shortest LOS had supplementary beds serving the district in another unit. This compares with only one of the eight hospitals with the longest LOS. In most cases, this means that longer-stay and more difficult patients can be transferred out of these units, which probably accounts for the small number of patients staying more than 6 months in these units.

Figure 3 shows that variation in the percentage of patients discharged in 1 or 2 weeks makes only a slight contribution to the unit's tendency to have a longer or shorter average LOS, as shown in Fig. 2. The data on this figure are also given in Table XIV, p. 37, columns F and G, but these refer only to the study of 400 discharges at the hospitals studied, and do not relate to all beds in the districts which have acute-case beds elsewhere (indicated by an asterisk).

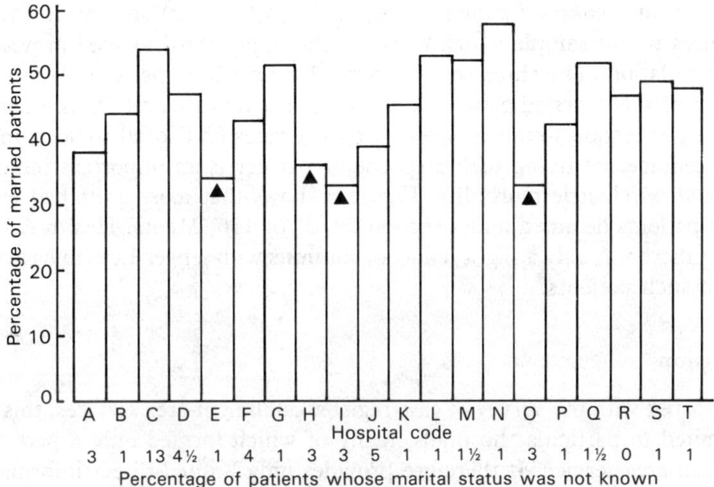

Fig. 5   Percentage of married patients by hospital. Hospitals marked ▲ have the lowest proportion of currently married patients and are in the districts with the highest bed provision and social morbidity indices. Hospitals are ranked by 'length of stay' as in Fig. 2.

Figure 4 and Table XIV show the percentage of discharged patients who were aged over 65 in these hospitals, and the percentage of the over-65s who stayed more than 6 months. These figures may include both ESMI and functionally ill over 65s, if they are occupying acute-case general psychiatry beds. Fig. 3 illustrates the importance, when planning, of distinguishing the special groups who occupy acute-case beds, since they make a significant contribution to the bed use (up to 52% of beds in some hospitals). However, the percentage of patients over 65 does not explain the variation in LOS between units shown in Fig. 2, which also shows the LOS after over-65s are taken out, for those hospitals that do not transfer patients or have a second unit in the district. Generally, the percentage of over-65s in acute-case units does not contribute to the variation between hospitals, because the proportion is fairly constant, but where there are excessive numbers over 65, this can markedly increase the LOS, and can be a key factor in some areas, e.g. hospital K, Figs 2 and 4.

Figure 5 shows that the percentage of unmarried patients in the unit does not account for differences in the acute-case LOS, but the four units with the highest

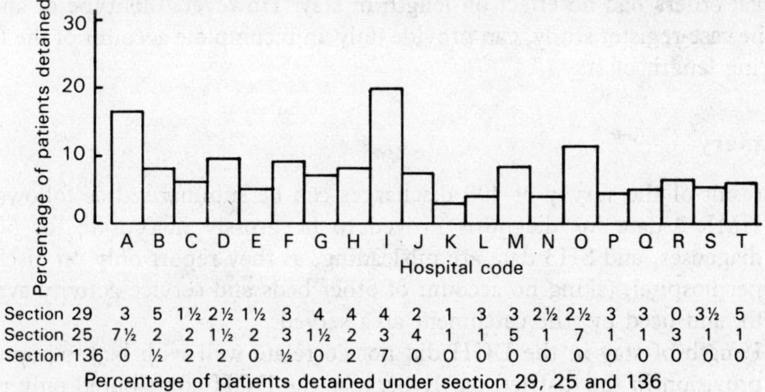

Fig. 6   Percentage of patients detained compulsorily.

proportion of *unmarried* patients (hospitals E,A,I and O) are within the group of services in our sample which make up the upper third for bed provision per 1000 population. The three services with the most beds per population all had less than 35% of married patients in their main acute-case unit. This is consistent with the correlation found between discharge rates and social indices, in which the percentage not living with a spouse or partner is an important indicator of social and psychiatric morbidity. Figure 6 shows that most units had less than 10% of patients detained under section 29, 25 or 136 (Mental Health Act 1959), and that there was only a slight tendency for units with longer LOS to have slightly more of such patients.

Discussion

As compared with the survey of case-register catchment-area services, this survey was limited to particular hospitals, many of which formed only a part of their catchment-area service. It therefore provides only limited direct information to explain the variation between districts in their bed-per-population ratios. However, it does provide useful background data for the further study of bed use in the respective catchment areas, as well as useful data about the operation of the individual units, the proportion of patients staying more than 3 or 6 months, and the factors which affect their length of stay and bed use.

In contrast to the survey of 20 hospitals and services described below, this survey dealt with all patients discharged from the acute-case general psychiatric unit, regardless of their age or place of residence, but excluding patients discharged after a year or longer of hospital stay. The data give a more realistic indication of the way in which DGH units work, especially since the hospitals were originally selected because they were thought to provide all the beds for their areas.

This survey confirms the key role of relatively few patients with an extended length of stay in determining bed use; they are an important factor in increasing acute-case bed requirements (Hirsch, 1983). On the other hand, the hospitals with an apparently short length of stay and high throughput usually had a supplementary unit to which they could pass on their patients with difficult problems. Bed use might have looked very different for these hospitals if they had not had a back-up hospital. The survey also showed that the percentages of over-65s and of currently unmarried residents may influence length of stay, but that the percentage of patients on legal orders had no effect on length of stay. However, this type of analysis, like the case-register study, can provide only an incomplete account of the factors affecting length of stay.

Summary

The result of the survey of 400 discharges can be summarised as follows:
1. HMR-1 data for diagnosis proved to be grossly inaccurate for 50% of diagnoses, and SH3 data are misleading, as they report only on discharges per hospital, taking no account of other beds and service activity available to, and used by, the catchment area served.
2. Length of stay in the DGH did not correlate well with bed-to-population provision in the district, partly because the DGH contributed only part of the total beds used in eight out of 20 districts studied ($r=0.21$).

3. Patients staying more than 6 months make a considerable contribution to the differences between hospitals on their average length of stay. However, five of the eight hospitals with the shortest length of stay had a supplementary unit, which accepted admission or transfer, e.g. of the longer-stay patients (Fig. 2).
4. Differences in the proportions of patients discharged within 2 weeks make only a small contribution to the variation in length of stay (Fig. 4 and Table XIII).
5. The proportion of patients over 65 varied between 12 and 50% of acute-case bed occupancy, but differences between hospitals in the percentage of over-65s did not account substantially for the variation in length of stay, except in a few cases, which had the highest proportion of patients aged over 65.
6. A high proportion of unmarried patients (over 35%) was associated with a longer length of stay.

5 Survey of hospitals and services by questionnaire and on-site consultation

The focus of this survey was the service provided within a catchment area for its population, after eliminating the effect of cross-boundary inflow. The working party tried to evaluate what was provided, and how well and to what extent it worked. As this report deals with planning for acute-case DGH units, elderly demented patients (ESMIs) and their service needs are not included. Information was collected on each of the 20 services. This consisted of a mixture of routine statistics, special data-gathering exercises and interviews with key personnel involved in the provision of psychiatric services. With the help of Dr D. Dick, then Director of the Health Advisory Service, an exhaustive list was compiled of the components of a comprehensive psychiatric service (Appendix 2). Using this list, a set of questionnaires (A to F) (available from Professor Hirsch) was prepared for the survey, which covered the following four main elements: (a) the characteristics of the catchment area and its population; (b) the characteristics of the hospital-based psychiatric services available to and used by the catchment area as a whole (questionnaires A,D,F); (c) the characteristics of social-services, voluntary and private facilities available to and used by the catchment area for the care of the mentally ill (questionnaire B); (d) the characteristics of the operating policies of the short-stay psychiatric unit (questionnaire D).

Methods

District health-service provision was first assessed by a questionnaire (A), which was sent to the District Medical Officer, prior to each visit; he was asked to define the acute-case-unit catchment-area population and the level of mental-health-service resources currently available to it. In the event, only half of the districts provided adequate information, but this was supplemented as necessary by a member of the research team, in consultation with personnel based at the unit at the time of the visit.

Social-services provision was assessed by sending a questionnaire (B) to the Director of Social Services; this covered the nature and extent of support services provided by the local authority, social services, voluntary and private agencies. However, as the response to it was so poor, questionnaire B was sent to the principal hospital social worker to be completed partially prior to the visit, and so to form the basis of a structured interview when the visit took place.

The information from these questionnaires and the results of the survey of 400 discharges were analysed for each hospital prior to the visit, and a supplementary information sheet (questionnaire E) was prepared to deal with unresolved issues which needed to be explored. Questionnaire E was used with questionnaire D (dealing with operating policy) as a basis for a semi-structured interview carried out by the research visitor with all the consultant psychiatrists associated with the acute-case unit. This also dealt with some of the wider issues connected with the provision of psychiatric care in the locality.

The nursing view was obtained from an interview, based on questionnaire F, with a senior nurse or nursing officer associated with the psychiatric unit at each hospital. After the visit, the interviewer completed a general impression sheet, and a questionnaire A feedback sheet, to check that the figures and information provided on questionnaire A tallied with the understanding obtained from the visit.

The survey of 400 patient-discharges concerned those during 1981. The questionnaires were sent out during 1982, and hospitals visited between October 1983 and August 1984. Efforts were made throughout to gauge the effect of policy changes on resources since 1981, in order to explain differences in the present resources since 1981 (Hirsch, 1983). Temporary changes, such as closing wards for upgrading, were ignored, and this is one of several factors which limit the accuracy of the data.

Visits to hospitals

This part of the survey was carried out with the collaboration and assistance of the Health Advisory Service (HAS), which provided three senior psychiatrists, experienced in making HAS visits, to carry out the survey visits. One HAS psychiatrist visited each hospital, except the first; in order to standardise the working party's approach, this was visited by all three, plus the Chairman and Mr H. Malin from the DHSS, who did the background work for each visit.

Information was collected before each visit and a member of the research team was briefed. The visitor sought further information to clarify and correct what had already been collected; he then carried out a semi-structured interview with key members of the consultant, nursing, social work, and junior medical staff.

General observations and results on the survey returns

As might be expected from a study of this type, the data were of variable quality. Even when dealing with identical aspects of the psychiatric service in a given locality, it was not uncommon to find that sources conflicted, and it was extremely difficult to obtain data that were consistent. At times, a 'best estimate' of the facts had to be made. Therefore, interpretation of some of the low correlations observed must take account of the fact that the quality of the data allowed for more error than was acceptable.

Definition of reference populations and services

The beds, services and needs of the catchment areas of the chosen units were the focus for this part of the study, but these were 'defined' catchment areas, as officially designated for each of the units, and were not necessarily identical with what might be described as the 'natural catchment areas' from which patients came. Adjustments for cross-boundary flows and outflows to other units are described below.

There were a number of complications surrounding the definitions of the designated catchment areas: of the 20 localities covered in this report, only eight had catchment areas which corresponded with health-district boundaries – either before the 1982 reorganisation of the NHS or after. Nevertheless, the catchment-area population, the service and the district are referred to here as if they referred to the same planning entity. Population figures which were used to determine resource-level-per-1000-population are for 1981.

Correspondence of reference catchment areas to social-service departments

As far as the linkage between the catchment areas and social service departments (SSDs) was concerned, only four corresponded to a single SSD, two to two SSDs, and two to three SSDs. The remaining ten catchment areas did not correspond to their associated SSDs, and in three of these catchment areas, four different non-corresponding SSDs were involved. In addition, the catchment areas of hospital 12 (Tables XII–XXIII) and hospital 10 were altered as a result of the 1982 reorganisation of the NHS, while another hospital also appears to have been catering for a different catchment area in 1986–1987, although the officially designated catchment area had yet to change. There was difficulty in establishing some of the main attributes of the populations involved, and hence the working party used no more than the most basic population data relating to all catchment areas, namely the total population and the proportion aged over 65.

Identifying and defining acute-psychiatric-case bed provision

The main problem in determining levels of acute-case bed provision is how to extract, in a consistent and meaningful manner, the confounding effects of those aspects of psychiatric in-patient care not included by the DHSS as acute-case general psychiatry – those concerning children, adolescents, ESMIs, and certain specialised facilities such as alcoholic units. Patients with stays of more than 1 year, and those treated in specialised units, are easy to identify; the elderly with mental illness present more of a problem. ESMI patients were defined as elderly patients with chronic irreversible confusional states. If beds were separately designated as ESMI beds, they counted as such, even if they might have been used for non-demented patients. However, there were instances when the elderly were being treated in acute-case wards; where this could be assessed, beds were discounted if they were used mainly for the ESMI.

Calculation of average and range of bed-to-population ratios as observed in 20 DGH services

Current level of beds for adult acute-case psychiatry
The first task was to determine, as closely as possible, the true number of acute-case general psychiatric beds available for each catchment area, and then to look at the factors which might account for the variation between areas in beds per population. The adjustments made to determine a standardised number for the acute-case general-psychiatry beds provided in each catchment-area service are shown in Table XIII, p. 24. Starting with the number of designated acute-case general-psychiatry beds (column C), the numbers of beds used for ESMI assessment were determined at the time of the working party's visits (column D), and an estimate was obtained of the number of beds occupied by new and established long-stay patients (column E). These were subtracted from the number of designated acute-case beds, to determine the number used by acute-case adult psychiatry patients (column F). Adjustments were then made to remove beds used by patients from other catchment areas (inflows) (column G).

In addition, it was found that a number of severely ill patients were either admitted directly to beds elsewhere in the district, or were transferred to such beds after a period on the main acute-case unit, and these should be included in the total bed resource for the population. Therefore, an adjustment was made to include additional beds formerly used by the district in hospitals other than the one visited (column H – outflow adjustment). In fact, five hospitals had a substantial bed supplement in other hospitals, and in one service, half the catchment-area work was done in another hospital. A few difficult patients were transferred to special units – these *ad hoc* arrangements were not accounted for, as the numbers were small and thought to be sporadic. Column H therefore represents the true adjusted estimate of acute-case general-psychiatry beds in use *within* the districts, but this does not include an estimate for patients having their treatment in *other* districts.

Cross-boundary outflow
Although an adjustment was made to exclude beds occupied by patients from other catchment areas, no adjustment was made for individuals from the catchment area who were directly admitted to hospitals outside their catchment area. A certain amount of cross-boundary flow occurs in almost all districts, such as to teaching hospitals and to hospitals just across the dividing line. If inflows are deleted without including an adjustment for cross-boundary outflows, there will be a systematic underestimate of bed needs. The outflow adjustment in Table XIII, column H, does not include cross-boundary flows; it only adds in supplementary beds run by the district in hospitals other than the one chosen for this study. The total number of resident cross-boundary inflow patients in the 20 hospitals deleted from column F to obtain column G is equivalent to 131 beds, or 9.9% of all acute-case beds in the 20 hospitals.

However, the distribution is skewed, with the inflow to eight hospitals averaging 20% (range 3–30%) and almost no inflow to the remaining 12. The figures in column N must therefore be increased by 10–20% to achieve an estimate of the overall true bed provision, if it is accepted that over a large number of districts, the overall cross-boundary outflow must equal inflow.

Beds per 1000 population provided for each catchment area
This figure is given in Table XIII, column J. It reflects the available acute-case
adult general-psychiatry beds provided by each health district (column H) for its
population, divided by the 1981 census figure for that district (column F). It does
not reflect the beds in use by the reference population, because cross-boundary
outflow is not included. This reflects provision and met demand, not 'need'.

The mean and median bed-per-population provision
The mean bed provision within the district per population ratio for the 20 hospitals
averaged from Table XIII, column J, is 0.37 (s.d.0.37±s.d.0.08) beds per 1000
population, with more than a three-fold difference between hospital 20 – with the
lowest provision, 0.16 beds per 1000 population and hospital 1 – with the highest
provision, 0.56 beds per 1000 population. The sample was skewed, and the median
was 0.395 per 1000. Although the observed range of bed use is 0.15–0.56 per 1000
population, other indicators must be examined, to decide if this provision is adequate
for the sample (discussed below). Adding 10% for cross-boundary outflow, the
figures are a mean of 0.41 per 1000 population and a median of 0.44 per 1000
population. The range in the sample is not as great as the range in the UK, which
is, at the very least, 0.12–0.76 beds per 1000 population, and possibly greater.

Discussion

These figures can be regarded as means and medians only for this sample, which
was stratified because the hospitals were chosen to reflect extremes of practice,
including hospitals with particularly high and low bed-turnover rates. Moreover,
the sample had a bias towards hospitals with higher bed-turnover rates (Table XII,
p. 23). Because the results are skewed, the median is a better indicator of the central
tendency than the mean, and provides a better basis for examining the factors which
may contribute to the variation in bed provision.

Even if the figures were a true reflection of bed provision in the hospitals studied,
there is a systematic underestimate of bed requirements, because cross-boundary
outflow has been excluded. Either cross-boundary inflow should not be excluded,
or an estimate for cross-boundary outflow must be included; otherwise, the group
of patients who go outside their district for treatment will be left out of the
calculations. The average should therefore be increased by 10%, but in planning
for a particular district, local conditions also need to be taken into account.

A judgement is required about whether there is a likely net inflow or outflow,
bearing in mind that the range of cross-boundary inflow for acute-case general
psychiatry varied from 0 to 20% in these 20 hospitals. How each district plans
for cross-boundary inflow and outflow remains a policy decision, but the patients
concerned need to be accounted for.

Consultants at five of the six hospitals with the lowest bed provision (those with
less than 0.30 per 1000 population) were dissatisfied with their current bed
provision, but when these consultants estimated the extra number of acute-case beds
they thought they needed for a satisfactory in-patient service, the increases would
not have been likely to push the average bed provision for this group much above
0.30 acute-case beds per 1000 population. On the other hand, consultants from
hospitals 1–13 with 0.37–0.56 beds per 1000 population (there were no hospitals

between 0.31 and 0.37) did not complain about their bed provision. Of the hospitals substantially above 0.39 per 1000 population (the median), the two highest are teaching-hospital units in large urban conurbations with a concentration of inner-city problems; the non-district aspect of their work is, of course, excluded. The hospital with the third-highest bed use had the highest proportion of elderly among all the localities visited, but both this hospital and the hospital ranked fourth may be overprovided for (see below).

To arrive at a best estimate of the mean, various adjustments can be made to the figures of bed provision. A recalculation of the mean bed-per-population ratio, omitting the hospitals just mentioned at the extreme bed-per-population ratios (below 0.30 or above 0.50), gives a mean of 0.38 beds per 1000 population, or 0.42 after a 10% adjustment for cross-boundary outflow. If all of those hospitals below 0.30 per 1000 population that were regarded by the consultants as having insufficient beds were given 0.30 beds per 1000 population, the mean for the 20 hospitals would be 0.40. The mean for the observed 20 hospitals was 0.37 – corrected for cross-boundary flow to 0.41; and the median was 0.395 – corrected to 0.44. The case-register study reported occupancy rather than available beds, but it picked up cross-boundary flows because it recorded bed occupancy of catchment-area patients, wherever they were admitted.

To operate an effective service, occupancy should be 80–90%, allowing for emergencies – an average of 85%; this means that 15% must be added to the reported observed occupancy, which was 0.39 for the case registers, yielding 0.46. Similarly, the figure estimated for beds occupied in England and Wales (Table X, p. 17) was 0.39, plus a 15% adjustment to allow for 85% occupancy, estimating the current norm for bed provision at 0.45.

Some estimates of current acute-case psychiatric bed provision

		Beds provided per 1000 population	
Table	*Source*	*Mean*	*Median*
Table XI, p. 18	England and Wales: All beds occupied < 1 year, age 0–64 (beds occupied 0.38/1000 plus adjustment)	0.447(A)	
Table VI, p. 15	Psychiatric Case Register: All beds, age 15–64 (occupied 0.38/1000 plus adjustment)	0.456(A)	
Table XIII, p. 24	20-hospital study: On-site 0.37% plus 10% cross-boundary flow	0.41(B)	0.44(B)
	Omitting extremes, 0.38 plus 10% cross-boundary flow	0.42(B)	

The above sets out various estimates of acute-case general-psychiatry adult bed use, based on the discussion above. These are averages with large ranges and standard deviations, but they reflect current practice, as estimated from three sources, and can be regarded as a starting point. 'A' refers to an allowance for 85% bed occupancy; 'B' indicates an adjustment for cross-boundary flow, which is estimated from an observed average inflow from other districts of 10%.

The working party concluded that the best estimate of current practice for determining local bed needs is 0.43–0.44 beds per 1000 population.

6 Factors affecting variation in bed use

A principal aim of this study is to identify factors influencing the range of bed use observed among hospitals and services, and to identify factors that planners can take into account when opting for a higher or lower bed provision. Tables XIV–XXI tabulate information from questionnaires A–F and the findings of the interviewers, as reported to the working party after visits to the 20 hospitals. These tables show the service provision and activity of the units, and give some subjective impressions obtained during local interviews with staff. Demographic data from the 1981 census, updated locally where possible, are also included. Special attention was paid to hospitals at the upper and lower ranges of bed provision, as it was hoped that this might help to highlight factors which differentiate between the two.

The overall conclusions are set out in the summary for this chapter, but it must be borne in mind that the data were based on the expressed opinions of hospital staff and on the conclusions of the visitor: epidemiological data were not generally available.

Characteristics of operational policy

Table XIX, p. 43 gives some information which reflects how different services operate. Columns D,E,F,G and I–L have already been commented on above in relation to the survey of 400 discharges. They deal with the key hospitals initially studied, not the total hospital facilities provided for each catchment area. Columns B and C reflect the findings about admission procedures for the 20 hospitals, as well as the consultants' views of the geographical distribution of the catchment area, in relation to each hospital. Special points in the admission procedure are highlighted in Table XIX, p. 43, column B, *but no pattern emerged to suggest that the presence or absence of a particular policy for dealing with potential admissions explained differences in bed use.*

Regarding the geographical relationship of the hospital to its catchment area, distance was a problem regarding access to the day hospitals in a few cases, but generally was not an important factor. The sample includes more hospitals with rural or mixed communities, e.g. hospital 12, which is located outside its catchment area. Two problems emerged in relation to hospitals at a distance from their catchment area: (a) certain patients required admission who might have done better in a day hospital; and (b) domiciliary visits were reduced

TABLE XIV
Factors reflecting bed operational policy

(A)	(B)	(C)	(D)	(E)	(F)	(G)	(H)	(I)	(J)	(K)	(L)	(M)
	Admission policy		Number of population >65 (1000's)	Percentage of population >65	Percentage discharged within 2 weeks	Percentage discharged within 1 week	Estimated percentage of beds occupied 6-12 months	Percentage of compulsory admissions by section			Percentage of married patients	Cross-reference to hospitals in Figs 2-6
	Hospital filter	Distance						Section 29	Section 25	Section 136		
1	OP department	Not a problem	28.32	16	50	30	3	1.5	2	0	34	E
2	N/A	No problem	28.86	15	39	24	2	4	3	7	33	I
3	Consultant +CPN	No problem	48.06	27	36	19	4	2.5	7	0	33	O
4	Some caution	No problem	16.94	18	42	23	5	1.5	2	2	54	C
5	Only for ESMI	Problem for day hospital	28.58	15	30	17	8	2.5	1.5	2	47	D
6	Through A&E	Some problem	32.03	17	56	33	2	5	1	0	48	T
7	CPN assessed	No problem	30.04	18	34	22	4	4	2	2	36	H
8	90% assessed	No problem	24.00	20	28	12	5	1	1	0	46	K
9	By consultant	No problem	32.76	14	46	20	5	2	4	0	39	J
10	CPN & consultants	Some problem	22.11	11	31	14	2	2.5	1	0	58	N
11	Admit to assess	Compact area	19.50	15	47	31	2	3	1	0	42	P
12	By consultant	10 miles from city	18.90	10	27	19	6	3	7.5	0	38	A
13	By consultants	No problem	28.77	16	42	28	6	4	1.5	0	52	G
14	Uses other hospitals	Problem for day hospital	70.29	15	35	22	4	3	5	0	53	M
15	A&E screening	No problem	37.53	13	52	35	3	3.5	1	0	49	S
16	By consultants & OPs	Irrelevant	33.55	14	30	20	—	5	2	0.5	44	B
17	By OP	Prevents DVs	24.63	14	42	27	—	3	1	0	52	Q
18	Pre-admission assessment	Irrelevant	41.00	15	38	22	—	3	3	0.5	43	F
19	By OPs & DVs	Problem	26.62	20	39	17	—	0	3	0	47	R
20	Pre-admission assessment	Close by	28.91	14	59	33	—	3	1	0	54	L

Columns D, and F–K are based on the survey of 400 consecutive discharges, and represent only the activity of the hospital visited, not of the combined catchment-area service.
LS=long-stay patients; CPN=community psychiatric nurse; A & E=accident and emergency; S=another unit; DVs=domiciliary visits; OP=out-patients; N/A=not applicable

because of distance and the non-productive time wasted by consultants in travelling. The overall effect may be to limit access and reduce the service, because more hospitals with distance problems are in the moderate- to low-use bands for bed use.

Day facilities

Table XV shows the range and extent of NHS day facilities, with comments. The number of places at each sub-unit is given in column A, and these are totalled and divided by the population, in thousands, to calculate the day-hospital provision per 1000 population shown in Table XXII, p. 52, column N. The ranked correlation between day-care places per 1000 population and bed provision is $r=0.44$, just significant at the $P \leqslant 0.05$ level. Table XIX, column B, shows the local-authority day-care provision. Of the 20 hospitals visited, five of the six units with the lowest bed provision were in the lower 50th percentile for day-care provision, and five of the six hospitals with highest bed provision were in the upper 50th percentile. Thus, *lower bed levels do not correlate with high day-care provision, and higher levels of beds do not correspond to low day-care provision. The units best provided with*

TABLE XV

Hospital-based day attendance facilities

Hospital	(A) Places (number attending site)	(B) Rehabilitation	(C) Acute cases	(D) Chronic cases
1	80 places	Some	Yes	About 1/2
2	100+25	Yes	Yes	Yes
3	Nil+75	Few	Few	Most
4	40+0	Yes	Yes	Yes
5	40+15	No policy	Poor use	About 1/2
6	50+60	Not defined	On-site	Peripheral
7	50 places	Some rehabilitation	Yes	Little
8	24+25	Through OTs	Poor use	Short term
9	50	Understaffed: thought not used to best advantage		
10	20	Not specific	Majority	Little
11	50 places	Mix of clients: Poor collaboration and design restrict use		
12	20+16	Off-site	—	All on site
13	22+26 Ind	Some	On wards	Mostly
14	30+180+50	Yes	Yes	Yes
15	35+50	Yes	Yes	Yes
16	80	Nursing shortage, hence no formal division of tasks		
17	50+6	Active	Few	Some
18	60+0	Some	Some	Some
19	0+40	Active in all three areas of work		
20	33+44	About 1/2	None	About1/2

Column A shows the number of NHS-provided day-hospital places; where there is more than one facility, the size of each unit is given, e.g., Hospital 2; 100+25, means Hospital 2 has a day hospital in two localities with a total of 125 places

The number of day places per 1000 population is given in Table XXII (column N) and local-authority provision is shown in Table XIX (column B)

Chronic cases=in-patients more than 1 year

Section 29, 25, 136=Mental Health Act compulsory admissions

OT=Occupational therapy

Table XVI
Out-patients and out-patient department waiting lists

(A)	(B)	(C)	(D)	(E)	(F)	(G)	(H)	(I)	(J)
		Out-patients					Waiting policy		
Hospital	New	Total	Percentage new	New out-patients per 1000 population	All out-patients per 1000 population	Urgent WL	Other WL	Special features	Walk-in patient
1	3189	23 493	14	18.02	132.73	At once	2–3 weeks	Many second opinions	No
2	1600	11 700	14	8.32	60.81	?	2–6 weeks	Support	To unit
3	760	6879	11	4.27	38.65	At once	3–6 weeks	Support	No
4	214	3173	7	2.27	33.72	At once	4 weeks	Not stated	Via A&E
5	566	4578	12	2.97	24.03	?	3–10 weeks	Accelerated discharge	N/A
6	516	4907	11	2.74	26.05	?	2–3 weeks	Not defined	No: A&E
7	309	2706	11	1.85	16.71	At once	2–4 weeks	Some	No: via GP
8	316	2966	11	2.63	24.72	?	3 weeks	Full assessment	N/A
9	304	5058	6	1.30	21.62	At once	0–3 weeks	Seven wait on ward	One section only
10	616	9422	7	3.06	46.88	At once	?	Neurotic patients as out-patients	None
11	335	3778	9	2.58	29.06	At once	4–6 weeks	Not stated	Via A&E
12	281	2019	14	1.49	10.68	1 month?	1 month	Supportive	None
13	736	9316	8	4.09	51.81	At once	3 months	N/A	None
14	2122	16 687	13	4.53	35.61	At once	2–13 weeks	—	Via A&E
15	532	3550	15	1.84	12.30	At once	1–12 weeks	Assessment and support	None
16	794	5279	15	3.52	23.39	A&E	3 weeks	GP & CPN	Via A&E
17	834	3630	23	4.74	20.64	At once	1–5 weeks	Pressured	N/A
18	391	4886	8	1.43	17.88	At once	6 weeks	Avoid admission	Via A&E
19	220	1680	13	1.65	12.62	At once	4 weeks	Some seen at DH	Via out-patients' department
20	525	9069	6	2.54	43.92	At once	3 weeks	Avoid admission	Via A&E

WL=waiting list; DH=day hospital; A&E=accident and emergency; N/A=not applicable *beds tend to be better provided with a variety of types of day-care facilities, and those with least beds are generally least provided with such facilities.*

Out-patient services

Out-patient activity and waiting policy for out-patients is examined in Table XVI. Hospital 1 (a teaching hospital), and hospitals 2, 10, 13, 14 and 20, have disproportionately high total out-patient activity in relation to their beds. Hospital 1 has a very large cross-boundary flow, which makes up for 38% of its bed use. However, although bed levels were corrected for cross-boundary flow, out-patient figures were not. If hospitals 1 and 20 (the highest and lowest) are excluded, there is a positive and significant correlation between high out-patient activity and high bed provision ($r=0.53$). Hospital 17, with a high proportion of new out-patients, has the only really rural catchment area, but its load of both new and established out-patients is not excessive in respect to population size; it appears to see more patients only once, probably because of the distance patients have to travel.

An active out-patient service tends to go with high rather than low bed use, while the opposite would be predicted if the out-patient service made up for low bed provision. Like day-care provision, *out-patient activity tends to parallel bed provision, although hospitals 10, 12, and 20 are exceptions, with heavy out-patient activity,* but fewer beds (columns E and F), so that the overall correlation of out-patient provision with beds per population is positive ($r=0.46$), which is just significant at the $P\leqslant 0.05$ level.

Medical and nursing staff

The number of consultants in each hospital is given in Table XVII, column B, and the ratio of population per consultant in Table XXII, column K. The mean size of the population per consultant correlated inversely with the beds-per-population ratio – the Spearman product–moment correlation – is -0.76, but the population-to-consultant ratio did not correlate significantly with the discharge rate ($r=0.33$). *The correlation between bed provision and consultant provision is the strongest relationship of bed levels to any other service variable examined.* Services which are well provided with one are well provided with the other; the link may mean that more consultants create more beds and out-patients, but not more admissions – insofar as there is no correlation between discharges and consultants.

Possibly, a decision to improve the consultant-to-population ratio is a strong indication of an intention to expand the total resources of the service: additional facilities tend to follow. However, it is also likely that the decision to expand the service occurs because of local recognition that current services are insufficient for the potential demand.

Nursing

There was no clear relationship between bed ratios and aspects of the nursing service (Table XVII) on the wards or in the community, except that, again, districts better

TABLE XVII

Consultants, nurses, and community psychiatric nurses (CPNs)

(A)	(B)	(C)	(D)	(E)
			Nursing	
Hospital	Number of consultants	Ward level	CPNs	Use of CPNs
1	11 (Teaching)	Not enough, consultants can be dismissive	6 CPNs to 248 patients	Limited by consultants' policies
2	5 (Teaching)	Good	11 CPNs to 500 patients	Flexible; GP + SW + consultants
3	4	Pleased with role	8 CPNs to 4850 patients	Liaise between consultant + GPs
4	2	Adequate	3 CPNs to 145 patients	Consultant attached
5	4	Consultant-sharing impairs effectiveness	13 CPNs to 416 patients	In clinical teams + nurse therapists
6	4	Good standard	2 CPNs to 98 patients	CPNs support mainly at primary health-care level
7	5 (General psychiatry)	Under pressure, day assessment valued	20 CPNs each to 50 patients	Two per consultant, rest to GPs
8	3	Get job satisfaction	3 CPNs to 204 patients	Assess; medicate; maintain
9	5	High quality	4 CPNs to 158 patients	In therapeutic and clinical team
10	3	Satisfactory	4 CPNs to 580 patients	40% of time to psychogeriatrician
11	2	Fair; low tolerance of behaviour problems	5 CPNs to 250 patients	Not satisfactory 1.5 per sector per consultant
12	3	Barely enough for therapeutic effect	10 CPNs in community	Community orientated with GPs
13	2 (Need +4)	Only adequate for routine work	5 CPNs each to 40 patients	Consultant dominated
14	6	Absence of sectors lowers efficiency	12 CPNs to 700 patients	CPN sectorised but not consultants
15	4 (Need +1)	OK; pressure on male wards	6 CPNs to 300 patients	Supportive with consultants
16	4	Inability to recruit nurses	4/5 CPNs to 345 patients	Support groups, clubs, home visits
17	3	High-quality EMSI pressure	3 CPNs to 159 patients	Follow-up in geographical areas
18	3	Satisfactory; quality improving	3 CPNs to 600 patients	Hospital based; to all consultants
19	2	Good job satisfaction	6 CPNs to 200 patients	Three per consultant; with GPs and social workers
20	3 (1 in post)	High quality; given responsibility	5 CPNs to 150 patients	Hospital based; sectorised; good

SW = social worker

provided with beds were also better provided with community psychiatric nurses (CPNs), measured in terms of the numbers of CPNs per unit population (shown as population in 1000s per CPN in Table XXII, p. 52, column I). Generally, morale was high in the nursing staff at all ranges of bed use, but more so where the bed population provision was highest or lowest.

Multidisciplinary teams (Table XVIII) may or may not operate at each level of bed ratios; they may not include consultants, but multidisciplinary teams are consistently present in the lowest-bedded services, which is likely to be a result of having to work at low ratios of beds and medical staff. When this occurs, medical staff are more likely to share responsibilities with nursing and social-work staff in order to keep even a minimal level of service operational.

TABLE XVIII
Functioning of multidisciplinary teams

(A) Hospital	(B) Operation	(C) Comment
1	A+ ward level	Very varied approach in large unit
2	Good	CPN backbone of community service
3	Work well	Very good consultant support and use of SWs
4	Good	See no need for sectorisation
5	Mostly paramedics	SW and OTs have little input to service
6	Not well developed	Slow to develop community-orientated service
7	OK, at ward level	GPs involved only at primary care level
8	Effective	Impressive input from psychology department
9	Present	One sector ahead of other three
10	Works well	Regular input by psychologists and OTs
11	Fair only	Too easy access to other Hospital; "Dumps" problems
12	Mixed opinions	One ward very good; others have problems with consultants
13	At ward level, OK	Old fashioned consultant-dominated service
14	Good relationships	Absence of sectorisation decreases efficiency
15	Not formally set up	Disciplines work well together
16	Hospital only	Much change 1981–1984
17	High quality	Working in key clinical areas; good service
18	Very limited	CPN sectorised but not consultants
19	Good, very effective	Very successful, with excellent community relationships
20	Good	No junior doctors, good relationships.

Mostly paramedics = only doctors, nurses and psychologists hospital-based, not social workers (SWs) or occupational therapists (OTs)

Community facilities and support

Table XIX shows the level of community support (columns B–E) and community-orientated aspects of the service (columns F–H). A consistent pattern emerges of worse facilities in the ten hospitals with lowest bed provision and of better facilities in the ten with the best provision, but there are both poor and well-provided services at every level. Thus four services with very limited numbers of *day-centre* places are among the lower ten, and three are among the upper ten; the same figures of four and three, respectively, apply to the availability of *residential care. Social-work support* can be calculated per 1000 population for hospital-based social workers, but not for community-based workers, because they tend to work on a generic model as part of a social-work team which has only some psychiatric responsibility. Social-work provision seems to be evenly spread throughout, with some services better

TABLE XIX
Community facilities? Social workers? Ease of discharge? Domiciliary visits

(A)	(B)	(C)	(D)	(E)		(F)	(G)	(H)
		Community facilities and support						
Hospital	Day hospital	Residential	SW (Hospital)	SW (Community)	1000 population/ hospital SW	Discharge	Domiciliary visits (DVs)	Domiciliary visits per 1000s population
1	60 places	60+58+22+16	7 full-time	4+3 general hospital SW	25	Usually quick	458	2.59
2	Well developed	Fair to good	6 full-time	Some	32	—	89	0.46
3	30 places	28+3=140	1 day hospital+ 1 rehabilitation	1 per team	89	Only a week	790	4.44
4	Inadequate	Very few	6.2 WTE	Generic	15	High support	89	0.92
5	30 places	Poor 0+7+16	3 full-time, 4 part-time	2 sp SW	42	9 waiting	450	2.36
6	None	3+6+31	1+1 generic	3 in teams	94	Impeded	659	3.50
7	30 places	6 group homes	4 full-time, 2 part-time	2	37	To West Park	159	0.95
8	20 places	7 Vol+PTIII	3	1 per area	40	SW helps	315	2.63
9	30 places	9+6+6	Total 7	Generic	29	Traditional	1250	5.34
10	6 used per annum	2+21+4	2 full-time	2 sp SW	100	SW assistant	500	2.49
11	Fair	Fair	4 full-time	Generic	32	Slow especially aged	500	3.85
12	None ?	6+3+8	2 in 3 teams	Minimal	95	30 waiting	257	1.36
13	20 places	6 group homes	4 full-time	2PSW	45	Wait on ward	400	2.22
14	Fair	Difficult	3 full-time	Generic	156	Slow	567	1.21
15	40 places	22+11+13	7.5 full-time	4 SSW	38	Good support	400	1.39
16	Limited SSD	Limited	N/K	Generic	N/K	Clubs and visits	127	0.56
17	None (local authority)	7+4+PTIII	5 SW	2 sp SW	35	Slow	230	1.31
18	Very limited	Very limited	3 full-time	Generic	91	6 month–1 year discharge	221	0.81
19	45 places	6+3+land ladies	3 SW/team	Generic	44	Good support	200	1.50
20	Very limited	Very limited	1 only	Generic	207	Limited support	561	2.72

Numbers 28+35+10, etc., indicate number of places at each facility.
PSW=psychiatric social worker; SSW=Social Services social worker; WTE=whole-time equivalents; N/K=not known; PTIII=Part III accommodation; gh=general hospital; sp=specialised

TABLE XX

Division into sectors, perceived needs and morale

(A)	(B)	(C)	(D)	(E)	(F)
			Satisfaction/working morale		
Hospital	Division into sectors	Needs	Beds	Day hospital	Team spirit
1	No	Double day places; more CPN; ward poor	Enough, need hostel provision	Need many more places	Patchy; nurses often unable to develop
2	Satisfactory	Intensive day-care+drug-abuse unit +community facility	Adequate but . . .	Too few places	Good
3	Two satisfactory	More day places; more CPN	Enough	Need acute-case places	Very good
4	Not needed	Psycho-geriatric+day hospital+day care +residential	Adequate but . . .	Dissatisfied	Good
5	In two sectors	More day care+hostel+EMSI beds	Increase to 100	Unsatisfactory	Underdeveloped
6	None	More CPN+day hospital+long stay	Surplus beds	Unsatisfactory	Not in evidence
7	Not on wards	More group homes & young-person hostels	Adequate when W.Pk included	Need more places	Very good
8	None	More hospital & community facilities	Need 8–10 for disturbed	Satisfactory	High-quality consultant lead
9	Yes	Improve joint plan+day care & residential	Pressure/adequate case	Need better provision	1 sector ahead of other 3
10	Yes	Major expansion both hospital & residential	Adequate acute-case	Provision needed in community	Satisfactory; high nurse input
11	Satisfactory	Psycho-geriatric service+day hospital+ residential	Enough; need psycho-geriatric beds	Limited	Fair
12	Yes by ward	Day hospital+nurses+SW support+ residential	Thought adequate	Grave shortage	1 ward good; 2 wards bad
13	None	Few, possibly more hostel places	Adequate never blocked	Need more places	OK: under senior-consultant pressure
14	Not yet	Day hospital+day care+residential+ psycho-geriatric	Adequate but . . .	Deficient	Fair: good relationships
15	No	CPN+beds+day hospital+consultant	Need 6 acute-case	Need more places	Good; design also good
16	Totally sectorised	Community facilities, day-care psycho-geriatric beds	Need more psycho-geriatric	Too small	Nursing shortage
17	No	Psycho-geriatric beds+day care	Not enough	Poor provision	High quality, high morale
18	Incomplete	Community facilities+day hospital+day care+residential	Adequate but . . .	Too few places	Poor in 1981
19	Total	More beds, more CPN	Not quite satisfactory	Adequate	Very good
20	Works poorly	More of all but keep balance	Too few	Too few places	Varied, generally good

Clinical psy=Itinerant psychiatric problems of young people

and others less adequately covered at almost every level. Paradoxically, discharges are held up in more of the hospitals with low bed provision than high provision; again, comparing the lower with the upper ten, the consultants in four hospitals with the lower number of beds complained of a slow patient-discharge rate, but only three in the better-provided hospitals did so, probably because rapid patient-discharges are more important to hospitals with the fewest beds. It supports the interpretation that because these hospitals are underbedded, the staff find that they cannot get the patients discharged quickly enough to meet their bed needs. Thus *these findings are contrary to the hypothesis that the hospitals which depend least on beds are able to do so because they have better community facilities.*

Only one sector of one hospital had a specially organised *walk-in service*, but several others were accessible through the casualty department, which appears to be more common among the hospitals with fewest beds. The domiciliary services were slightly more active among the lower bed users, and were felt to be helpful in reducing admissions. The number of *consultant domiciliary visits* (DVs) is probably not accurate, but varied from 0.56 per 1000 population to 5.3 per 1000 population per annum. However, hospital 1 (highest in bed provision) had 2.6 per 1000 population per annum, and hospital 20 had 2.7 DVs per 1000 population, the mean for all 20 hospitals being 2.5 per 1000 population per annum. *Thus, DVs do not correlate with the variation in bed use.*

Table XX (column B) shows that more than half the hospitals, both in the upper and lower rankings for beds-per-population ratio, are *not split into sectors. The existence of sectors is independent of bed use.* Column C summarises what the consultants perceived as their service's greatest needs. There was a widespread request for more day-care facilities at all levels, as well as for more residential places to which patients could be discharged, and for more support staff. Hospitals ranked 8, 10, and 20 wanted 'more of everything', but there was no perceived need which distinguished those with high from those with low bed provision.

TABLE XXI

Characteristics of the population as described by staff

Hospital	Population type	Social status
1	Urban	Mixed, poor areas predominate
2	Urban	'Inner city' factors + high illegitimacy
3	Urban	'Itinerant psychiatric problems' + many aged people
4	Mixed	'New Town' + rural + above average income
5	Mixed/urban	Supportive community + affluent/aged people
6	Mixed	Relatively high proportion of aged people
7	S-E commuter	Supportive, accept psychiatric services
8	Mixed	?Psychiatric morbidity of Yorkshire Dales
9	Urban	Relatively static population
10	Mixed	Areas of high unemployment
11	Mixed	London suburb but few 'city' problems
12	Urban W-Midlands	Limited support; 'city' factors
13	N industrial	Some poverty; no 'city' factor
14	Mixed	Very high unemployment in towns
15	N Mining	Stable mixed N community
16	Outer London borough	Some middle-class people + inner-city problems
17	Rural	Some London overspill + forces
18	Mixed	High unemployment + immigrant people
19	Rural	Stable: rural with small towns
20	Urban	Mining community, supportive, high level of local identity, high unemployment

Dissatisfaction was experienced by all hospitals with a ratio of 0.3 per 1000 beds or less, but only four of them were felt by the local consultants to need more beds. The least-bedded service (hospital 20) had less than half the mean number of beds of the other three. If the four hospitals who expressed a need for more beds were to be given what they wished, the average bed-level provision for the 20 hospitals would be above 0.40 per 1000 population. Although there was widespread dissatisfaction with the quality of day-hospital provision, team spirit was not judged by our visitors to be different between high- and low-bedded districts.

Table XXI shows various characteristics of the population as perceived by hospital staff, which were thought possibly to be important in determining perceived demand. No type of population group – rural against urban, industrial against non-industrial etc. – related to high or low bed use. High unemployment occurred at all levels, as did the urban factor. However, these observations were based on the consultants' opinions, not statistical assessments.

Finally, the quality of the information available on suicide rates was insufficient to draw any conclusions.

Summary

There was no confirmation of the hypothesis that services with fewer beds per population would be compensated for, or complemented by, other NHS facilities. In fact, the visitors' impression was that shortages were observed in every aspect of the ancillary services, so that no such correlations could be expected. There was either no relationship between support services and bed use, or else a trend for those with fewer beds also to have fewer day-hospital and day-centre facilities, fewer consultants, fewer out-patient visits, fewer nurses, fewer community psychiatric nurses, slower patient-discharge rate and worse community support.

In spite of some indication that hospitals with fewer beds had relatively more consultant domiciliary visits and direct-access to walk-in out-patient facilities, there was no consistent trend in the relationship of types of admission service to number of beds. Distance from the catchment area tended to result in poor access, and a poorer domiciliary service. Again contrary to expectation, discharge was perceived to be delayed more in the low-bedded services. This may be relative to their low bed levels, but it also reflects the poor level of community support in their districts, and is consistent with the finding that low bed provision is associated with low resources generally, and with slow turnover.

Despite the very considerable differences between the lowest and highest bed users, there were no special features or types of service which could explain the variation: a consistent impression was that very low bed provision reflected a generally impoverished service. Thus, the Health Advisory Service visitors who carried out the survey of 20 hospitals for this report thought that the level of resource provision was not sufficiently complete in any of the services to allow an adequate test of hypotheses (3) and (4) [p. 22] – that ancillary services provided by the local authority and a community-orientated psychiatric service compensate for and are inversely correlated with bed provision. A more correct interpretation, though, would be that the provision of ancillary and community-orientated services in the sample did not offer an explanation for the variation in bed levels observed, but this does not rule out the possibility that such a relationship would hold if alternative services were provided at a sufficiently high level.

7 Estimating bed use, efficiency, and bed needs

It is clear that districts and services vary in the quantity as well as the quality of service provided, although much depends on the reliability and validity of the measurements made. There are at least three major factors to be considered: the resources provided (and how they are provided); the extent to which they are used; and the need for them. Resources can be quantified in terms of those aspects of the service that the health authority pays for, including the number of beds, consultants, day places, etc, while use can be quantified in terms of the level of activity of the service – the number of discharges, patient contacts, etc. These may not reveal much about the quality of the service which, in any case, depends greatly on subtle human factors. But the resources available and the level of activity generated from them are essential ingredients; for a given level of demand the service may be anything from inadequate to over-and-above what is needed.

There is a large measure of agreement in the UK as to the elements of a good psychiatric service (see Appendix 2) and how they should be provided with a limited number of options; these include an in-patient service, day hospitals and day care, a domiciliary service by consultants and CPNs, etc. Discussions about where these are situated – in mental hospitals or DGHs, or in the community – and the extent to which other aspects of the service should be hospital- or community-based, vary according to local conditions and policies. The style of the service, how it is organised, and its success in dealing with problems also depend on the human factor, which will vary whatever the resource. *It is reasonable to quantify the resources and the level of activity as a ratio per 1000 population.* This gives planners a basis of comparison between services and between districts, which can be the starting point for judging how one service compares with others. Decisions can then be made as to what should and will be provided in the future, and in what form, according to the local interpretation of needs and priorities, and how these can best be met.

Efficiency, efficacy, and demand

A principal aim of a service is to meet the health needs of its population and to provide as good treatment as possible, given the current state of medical and psychiatric knowledge. There may be other aims, such as prevention and education, but these are not the concern here. The success of a service in meeting these aims will be called here the *efficacy*, and this can be distinguished from its *efficiency*, which, from a planning and management point of view, can be measured in output terms: what level of activity has been generated with a given quantity of resource. *Activity* depends on demand. If there is low demand (e.g. because the service is of poor quality), then the level of activity will be lower than if the service is good. Demand and activity are also dependent on the level of resources, because if the resources are inadequate in quantity or quality, demand will be low.

Morbidity, or potential demand

Although activity is a measure of met demand, how can the level of need or potential demand be gauged, and how can the amount of psychiatric morbidity in a catchment area be estimated? The investigation of the relationship between admission rates and social morbidity in Hammersmith and in the North West Thames Region (chapter 2) showed a strong correlation between patient-discharge rates and social indices.

In all, five studies showed that discharge rates varied with indicators of social deprivation, even when demographic areas studied were served by the same psychiatric service. A relationship can also be demonstrated between discharges and Jarman UPA scores across the 20 services which comprised the present study. Thus, social morbidity appears to be a good indirect indicator of both psychiatric morbidity and potential need, and is a better indicator than current met demand, which is dependent on the nature of the service provided. In Appendix 3 we set out a method for weighting the provision of beds and resources allocated to a district according to predicted morbidity as estimated by socio-demographic indices.

If this argument is accepted, then it could be useful to compare activity against resources in order to measure efficiency, as well as resources and activity against social morbidity, to see if the service adequately provides for the potential need and potential demand. The 20-hospital study shows how this approach can be adopted to plan for bed needs.

In the following section, a model is developed to determine a relative rating between districts of their service activity, resources, and potential demand, and the model is applied to the 20 hospitals in our study. This should be regarded only as a first attempt, which needs to be refined and extended, but as a model it does provide a way forward for the planning of psychiatric beds and resources in the NHS.

Calculating measures of activity: resources, and potential demand

The general approach is to create a table of standardised values or scores for each of the planning variables: activity, resources and potential demand. A standardised score is a way of measuring the extent to which any value, such as the number of beds or number of CPNs per 1000 population in a district, differs from its mean value, expressed as standardised units from the mean. The working party then adopted two thirds of the standard deviation of the mean for each variable as the standardised unit, and Table XXIII shows the number of standardised units each district has above (+) or below (−) the mean on each variable.

A weighting was assigned to the different variables, according to the importance we ascribed to them in contributing to the service, i.e. as major planning factors; a weighted summed score was then calculated for activity, resources, and potential demand. Thus, the working party regarded out-patient visits as four times more important than CPN visits (in terms of their place in the calculation of the activity or work accomplished by the service), but consultant domiciliary visits are weighted to the same degree as CPN visits. These may be regarded as *ad hoc* guesses of the relative weightings, but different systems that were tried appeared to have similar general effects.

In the future, it would be possible for every district to collect its own data, according to predetermined national criteria; these data could then be used to assess and compare districts' resources and activity. Agreement would need to be reached about the relative weightings. Depending on data available from most districts, a new set of factors should be further developed to calculate, respectively, the level of resource available, and the usage of that resource for each service.

Calculation of standardised scores and activity analysis

The weightings used in this formula are *ad hoc*, they are simply based on their apparent reasonableness or 'face validity'. With larger numbers and further research, they would almost certainly be modified. The variable number of patient-discharges per 1000 population can be used as an example of how to calculate a standardised score. The mean ($\pm$s.d.) (column E) shown in Table XXII is 3.18 ($\pm$1.35). A score is thus derived for each of the values for each hospital by calculating how far the value lies from the mean in terms of the number of standard units (here defined as equal to 0.66$\times$s.d.) above or below the mean. The scores on deviation from the mean are obtained by banding the results for activity and resource item (the bands are based on 0.66 of a standard deviation). Those hospitals where the variation from the mean is less than 1 score zero; where the variation is >1 but <2, a score of 1 is given; where the variation is >2 but <3, a score of 2 is given, and so on. The score is given an appropriate $+$ or $-$ value, depending on whether the value is more or less than the mean value. The standard unit for discharges per 1000 population is 0.66$\times$1.35, or 0.90. The standardised number of discharges per 1000 population for hospital 1 in Table XXII (column E) is the difference between 4.69 and the mean 3.19, i.e. 1.50 divided by the standard unit of 0.90, i.e. 1.67. It is thus in the band 'greater than 1 but less than 2' standard units from the mean: so that in Table XXIII, it is given a score of $+1$. Hospital 6 had 7.36 discharges per 1000 – a difference of 4.18 from the mean. Dividing 4.18 by 0.90 gives 4.64, or about 5 standard units. Hospital 16 has 0.98 discharges: $3.20-0.98=2.22$. Then, 2.22 divided by $0.90=2.47$, or, between 2 and 3 units *below* the mean – so that a score of -2 has been given in Table XXIII, as the value is below the mean.

After the standardised scores for each variable were determined, the weighted scores for each district service were calculated according to the formula:

Activity $=2\times$ discharge score $+2\times$ out-patient department
$+0.5\times$ DVs score

Had reasonable data been available, the formula would have been:

Activity = 2 × in-patient discharges score
            + 2 × out-patient department score + 0.5 DVs score
            + 0.5 × day hospital attendances score + 0.5 × CPN score.

The weightings were based on the reasoning that each hospital's patient-discharge rate represented a much greater concentration of clinical activity than its CPN or domiciliary visits. The total number of out-patient visits per 1000 population over a year varies from 10 to 132 per 1000 population, and the number of in-patient discharges from 1 to 7.4. As the standardised scores are an indication of how far a particular value varies from its mean, it does not reflect the amount of activity involved in an out-patient visit, CPN visit or an admission to hospital.

The weightings used for this report were based on an estimate of the amount of activity involved in, for example out-patients in total, compared with in-patients or DVs in total; they should try to take account of the total concentration of resources and amount of activity involved. For example, if there are 10–135 out-patient visits, compared with 1–7 discharges per 1000 population, this represents a 10- to 20-fold difference in the numbers. An out-patient visit is a single event, but an in-patient eventually discharged stays 38 hospital days on average and uses much staff time. The most valid weighting could probably be arrived at by an analysis of the *economic cost* of each variable in an out-patient visit on admission, etc. However, these data are not available.

The weighted standardised scores for activity are shown in Table XXIII, p. 54. This shows the weighted total score for each service above or below the mean. The score for hospital 1 is 12, and for hospital 20 it is −4. There is a distortion here, which reveals a problem in using these data. Although the number of occupied beds per 1000 population for hospital 1 has been adjusted for cross-boundary inflows (a reduction of 30%, the out-patient activity of hospital 1 has not been similarly adjusted – but it is much larger than in the other hospitals. Similar problems occur in other hospitals with high cross-boundary flows, if these are not adjusted when calculating rates for population at risk.

Another problem is that the data were not sufficiently accurate to include hospital day-visits in the activity analysis. The discharged patients per bed per service, and length-of-stay figures, were calculated indirectly, because it was necessary to use the percentage occupancy figures from SH3-1979 (the NHS bed-occupancy figures). These are not accurate for districts which have acute-case patients in more than one hospital, because the survey of 400 discharges was limited to one hospital in each district. The data for hospitals without outflow are more accurate; the discharge rates for hospitals 6,9,10,11,14,18, and 19 are therefore less reliable, because those units had a considerable outflow to other units in the district. Notwithstanding this limitation, meaningful correlations between patient-discharge rates and other variables were observed. More accurate data would improve the relevance of the model, but the data are sufficient for illustrative purposes.

Table XXII shows the activity of other aspects of the service and the hospitals' ranking on each factor. Table XXIII shows their standardised scores and the weighted totals. The weighting factors, based on best estimates, were checked against another system of weighting, whereby the hospitals were given points on each variable according to their ranking among the 20 hospitals. Each variable was weighted and the weighted sum calculated to give a total weighted ranking for activity and resources for each district service.

The six top-ranking hospitals on each variable were given three points, the middle ranking two, and the seven hospitals ranked lowest on any variable were given one point. The summed rankings were then used to create an activity and resource scale, which gave similar results to the standardised score method described above. The advantage of using standardised scores is that any hospital can calculate its own score in terms of standard units from the mean, and compare it with the results. For this reason, the working party chose to use the standardised score method.

Activity analysis provides a useful way of evaluating an important aspect of current practice: how much is going on in the service. Hospitals with the highest levels of activity tend to have the most beds, but hospitals 6,9,11, and 13 have high activity yet moderate or low bed numbers, and these would be the most efficient by our measures. Hospitals 4,5,7,12,14,16,17,18,19, and 20 have low activity, but only hospitals 4,5,7, and 12 have low activity in relation to a relatively high number of beds: they can be considered less efficient. Hospitals 12,15,16,18,19, and 20 run a generally lower level of service, with lower activity and low resources. By contrast, hospitals 1,2, and 3 have a high level of activity but also a high level of beds and resources. The analysis suggests that some services are inefficient – in the sense that there is a relatively low level of service provided in relation to the number of beds used for in-patient treatment.

Resources analysis

The total resource provided by the district can be estimated in a similar way, relative to all other health districts. The district's provision of beds, relative to the rest of the mental-health resources and relative to other districts, can also be evaluated. An example of how a weighted figure for resource can be calculated is:

$$\text{Resource} = 3 \times \text{beds}/1000 \text{ population} + 2 \times \text{consultant}/1000 \text{ population} + 1 \times \text{CPN}/100 \text{ population} + 1 \times \text{day places}/1000 \text{ population} + 0.5 \times \text{hospital and community-based SWs}/1000 \text{ population} + 0.5 \times \text{resident places}/1000 \text{ population} + 1 \times \text{out-patient sessions held} + 1 \text{ walk-in clinic service} + 1 \times \text{community day-centre services} + \text{etc.} = \text{total weighted resources score}$$

A simpler calculation was used because data for most of these factors were unavailable. The formula used in Table XXIII is:

$$\text{Resource} = (2 \times \text{beds}/1000 \text{ population}) + (2 \times \text{consultant}/1000 \text{ population}) + (0.5 \times \text{CPN}/1000 \text{ population}) + (0.5 \text{ day hospital places}/1000 \text{ population}).$$

The standardised score and weighted resource score for each district was then calculated. The results are shown in Table XXIII.

Morbidity analysis: social indicators of predicted demand

It is not feasible to carry out in-depth studies in every district or on a regular basis. Such an approach assumes unimpeded access to individuals and their homes at all levels in the community, as well as access to records of their personal state of mental health – something which can by no means be assumed. It also assumes

TABLE XXII

Activity and resource indicators of psychiatric services and their ranked order in the 20-hospital study

(A) Hospital	(B) Provision/ 1000 population	(C) Rank order of beds/population	(D) Population (1000s)	(E) Patient-discharges per 1000 population	(F) Rank order patient-discharges	(G) Number of CPNs	(H) Patients per CPN	(I) 1000 population/CPN	(J) Rank order of CPN per population
1	0.56	1	177.00	4.69	4	6	41	29.50	8
2	0.50	2	192.40	4.81	3	11	45	17.49	3
3	0.48	3	178.00	5.11	2	8	60	22.25	5
4	0.46	4	94.10	2.00	16	3	48	31.33	9
5	0.42	5	190.50	2.28	14	13	32	14.65	2
6	0.42	5	188.40	7.36	1	2	49	94.20	19
7	0.41	7	166.90	2.98	11	20	50	8.35	1
8	0.41	7	120.00	2.43	13	3	68	55.63	16
9	0.40	9	234.00	3.42	8	4	39	58.50	17
10	0.40	9	201.00	3.97	6	4	145	50.25	15
11	0.39	11	130.00	4.25	5	5	50	26	7
12	0.37	12	189.00	1.76	18	10	N/A	18.90	4
13	0.37	12	179.80	3.16	10	5	40	35.96	10
14	0.30	14	468.60	3.22	9	12	58	39.05	11
15	0.27	15	288.70	3.50	7	6	50	48.12	14
16	0.24	16	225.70	0.98	20	5	N/K	45.10	13
17	0.23	17	175.90	2.45	12	3	53	58.63	18
18	0.23	17	273.30	1.83	17	3	200	91.10	20
19	0.18	19	133.10	2.20	15	6	34	22.80	6
20	0.16	20	206.50	1.27	19	5	230	41.30	12
Mean	0.37			3.18				40.41	
0.66×s.d.	±0.06			±0.90				±13.6	

(Continued)

(K) 1000 population per consultant	(L) Rank order of population/ consultant	(M) Day-care places at Hospital	(N) Day hospital 1000 population	(O) Rank order of day-care places per population	(P) New OP/1000 population	(Q) All OP/1000 population	(R) Rank of all OP/population	(S) Domiciliary visits (DVs)	(T) Domiciliary visits (DVs)/ 1000 population
16	1	80	0.45	4	18.02	132.73	1	458	2.59
38.4	3	125	0.65	1	8.32	60.81	2	89	0.46
44.5	5	75	0.42	6	4.27	38.65	6	790	4.44
47	7	40	0.43	5	2.27	33.72	8	87	0.92
47.6	9	55	0.29	14	2.97	24.03	12	450	2.36
47.1	8	110	0.58	2	2.74	26.05	10	659	3.50
33.4	2	50	0.30	12	1.85	16.21	17	159	0.95
40	4	49	0.41	7	2.63	24.72	11	315	2.63
46.8	6	50	0.21	17	1.30	21.62	14	1250	5.34
67	15	20	0.10	20	3.06	46.88	4	500	2.49
65	13	50	0.38	8	2.58	29.06	9	500	3.85
63	12	36	0.19	18	1.49	10.68	20	257	1.36
89.5	19	48	0.27	16	4.09	51.81	3	400	2.22
78.1	18	260	0.55	3	4.53	35.61	7	567	1.21
72.2	17	85	0.29	14	1.84	12.30	19	400	1.39
54.42	10	80	0.35	10	3.52	23.39	13	127	0.56
58.6	11	56	0.32	11	4.74	20.64	15	230	1.31
91.1	20	43	0.16	19	1.43	17.88	16	2214	0
66.55	14	40	0.30	12	1.65	12.62	18	200	1.50
68.8	16	77	0.37	9	2.54	43.92	5	561	2.72
56.12			0.35			34.17			2.09
11.03			±0.08			±15.78			±0.79

N/A = not applicable; N/K = not known; OP = out-patient

TABLE XXIII

Standardised scores for activity and resource analysis

| Hospital | Weighting for activity | | | | | Resource weighting | | | | | |
| | Standard scores for | | | | | Standard scores for | | | | | |
	Beds/ population	Patient- discharges	O/P per 1000 population	Domiciliary visits	Weighted score for weighting	Beds/ population	Population/ consultant	Population/ CPN	D/C per population	C' places/ population	Weighted score for resources
1	3	1	5	0	12	3	3	0	0	0	12
2	2	1	1	−2	3	2	1	1	3	0	8
3	1	2	0	2	5	1	1	1	0	7	4.5
4	1	−1	0	−1	−2.5	1	0	0	1	0	2.5
5	1	−1	0	0	−2	1	0	1	0	0	2.5
6	1	4	0	2	9	1	0	−2	2	0	2
7	1	0	−1	−1	−2.5	1	2	1	0	0	6.5
8	0	0	0	0	0	0	1	0	0	0	2
9	0	0	0	4	2	0	0	−1	−1	0	−1
10	0	0	0	0	0	0	−1	0	−2	0	−3
11	0	1	0	2	3	0	−1	1	0	0	−1.5
12	0	−1	−1	0	−4	0	−1	1	−2	0	−2.5
13	0	0	1	0	2	0	−3	0	−1	0	−6.5
14	−1	0	0	−1	−0.5	−1	−2	0	2	0	−5
15	−1	0	−1	0	−2	−1	−1	0	0	0	4
16	−1	−2	0	−2	−5	−1	0	0	0	0	−2
17	−2	0	0	−1	−0.5	−2	0	−1	0	0	−4.5
18	−2	−1	−1	−1	−4.5	−2	−3	−3	−2	0	−12.5
19	−2	−1	−1	0	−4	−2	0	1	0	0	−3.5
20	−3	−2	0	0	−4	−3	−1	0	0	0	−8

This table shows the standardised score or number of standardised units of 0.66×s.d.: each score stands above or below the mean. The districts studied are indicated by the first column

Each standardised score equals $(0.66 \times \dfrac{\text{True value}}{\text{s.d. of mean}})$

OP=out-patients; D/C=discharges; C' places=community places

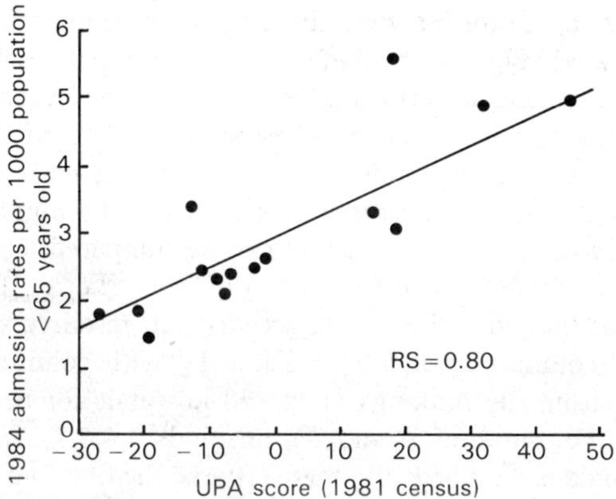

Fig. 7 Jarman Underprivileged Area (UPA) scores for districts of the North West Thames region.

unimpeded access to the service of those in need, but only one in eight or so of those with significant morbidity is referred to it (Goldberg & Huxley, 1980).

An indirect approach is to look at indices of social morbidity or deprivation, such as the Jarman Underprivileged Area (UPA) score, which has been found to be a good predictor of demand for psychiatric services.

The UPA score is a composite score of values for eight socio-demographic variables, using 1981 Census data; each variable is expressed as the percentage of the resident population characterised by the variable (except unemployed). The variables are: elderly living alone, under 5s, one-parent families, unskilled, unemployed, overcrowding, moved-home recently, and those born in the 'new Commonwealth' or Pakistan. The scores for the eight variables were normalised, standardised, weighted and summed to give a single global score of underprivilege for a population unit (e.g. electoral ward, DHA). The weightings were assigned to the variables from the results of a questionnaire sent to one in ten GPs in England and Wales (77% response rate). Jarman allowed the working party to include the UPA scores for the district health authorities of England as Appendix 1. Appendix 3 shows how they can be used to weight district bed and resource provision. For the 20 hospitals in this survey, the discharge rates and Jarman UPA scores of each hospital's district health authority correlated, $r = 0.41$ ($P = 0.05$). The correlations for Foster's study in Hammersmith and for the district of the North West Thames Region (see pp. 8, 9; Table V, p. 11, and Fig. 7) were considerably higher. However, the 20 hospitals varied considerably in resources, activities and style of services; furthermore, cross-boundary flow was not considered, and the UPA scores used were not those of the hospital catchment areas, but those of the district in which the areas were sited. The DHA and service boundaries coincided for only eight of the twenty hospitals.

Estimating appropriate needs

By combining and comparing a district's observed bed/population ratio and its relative ranking on the activity analysis, resources analysis, and social morbidity indicators, it is possible to form a view about the relative quantity and efficiency of the service provided. This can be done by comparing potential demand, based on the social morbidity index or Jarman UPA score, with the level of clinical activity of the service. In this way, if activity matches potential demand, one can examine activity and potential demand against the total resources committed to mental-health services for the population served, and against the number of beds.

Thus, levels of individual service factors can be compared, e.g. bed provision with an index of potential demand (column A of Table IV, p. 10, with either of columns F or G) or the global indices of activity and resource with an index of potential demand (columns D and E of Table IV with columns F or G). For example, by comparing the rankings of the 20 hospitals for bed provision and UPA score (Table IV, columns A and F), hospitals 3,4,5,7,13, and 18 may be inappropriately provided with beds. By these criteria, the first four have a relatively high bed provision, with relatively low UPA scores, and the latter two have low bed provision and high UPA scores. Besides having a high level of bed provision, hospitals 3,4,5, and 7 have a high level of resources and a comparatively low level of underprivilege. However, hospital 3 contrasts with the others, in that it provides an active service, whereas hospitals 4,5, and 7 are services with a low level of activity, either due to low demand or inefficiency. Hospital 8 is a good example of a service where activity, resources, and potential demand appear appropriately matched for the area. Hospital 16 is ranked near the middle for potential demand and resource, but the activity ranking is low, implying that the service provided is probably inefficient.

The four hospitals with the lowest bed provision make an interesting contrast. According to these measures, hospitals 17 and 19 have lowish UPA scores, but hospital 17 showed a fairly high level of activity, as well as low bed numbers. Hospital 17 appeared to provide a reasonably active service, relative to a low potential need and low bed provision; hospital 19, on the other hand, was providing a low level of service activity in an area of least need. That contrasts with hospital 18, which is high on UPA score but has the lowest of all the resource scores and a low activity score; this service was clearly underserviced, relative to potential demand. Hospital 13 is similar to hospital 18, in that it services an area of high deprivation and is underresourced, but in contrast to hospital 18, it provided an active service. Hospitals 1 and 2 are both teaching hospitals, with high levels of resource and activity, providing a high level of service in areas of high potential demand.

Obviously, policy decisions are affected by factors other than these measures. It may be thought inappropriate to increase resources for a service situated some miles from its catchment area, when the needs of the area are also being met by cross-boundary flow to a nearer service. The hospital receiving the cross-boundary flow would require resources in excess of those justified only by its catchment area's potential demand. These examples illustrate how the collection of simple data relative to the size and use of resources allows planners to gauge certain quantitative aspects of mental-health services which can be vital to planning for psychiatric beds.

8 An approach to planning for beds and resources

The working party has suggested an approach to planning that depends on the availability of routine data concerning a district's resources and the clinical activity generated by these resources; which can then be compared with various indicators of potential demand. Jarman's index of underprivileged areas is a good predictor of potential demand for the care of adult mental illness, and it may prove equally valid in other areas of psychiatric illness and health care, as well as in predicting the need for social services. Mortality data and other indicators of health care have been considered in relation to the Resources Allocation Working Party (1976), and may be more relevant to certain other kinds of health care.

The approach suggested here depends on the collection of descriptive data by health authorities about their services. It is consistent with, but goes beyond, the recommendations of the Korner Report (1982), and can be seen as a response to criticism of the Report of the Royal Commission on the National Health Service (1979; paras 21.56-21-60) on the dearth of information available for the monitoring and control of resource utilisation in the NHS.

If adequate data on resource provision (resources) and utilisation (activity) are available for each health district, comparison between districts is straightforward. The approach can be expanded and made much more detailed, and could, for comparison purposes, be simplified from the resource point of view by comparing financial expenditure on mental-health services across districts, per head of population served. However, it will be some time before such information will be available.

The close correspondence between bed use and data on bed provision, collected in this and in national and case-register studies, suggests that the 20 hospitals described here were reasonably representative of the DGH-based psychiatric services in England and Wales. Until a register is provided, though, showing the relative ranking by all districts in the UK for resources and activity, individual districts can analyse their local activity and resource following the example provided here. A more sophisticated approach would record all aspects of service provision and utilisation. All figures should be stated as rates per 1000 population in the district.

Data which should be routinely available from every health district:

> number of beds, sub-categorised for specialty units, ESMI, and children;
> length of stay, and number of discharged patients per bed per year;
> percentage occupancy in each category;
> information on cross-boundary flow;
> numbers of discharges and deaths;
> out-patients: first attendance (new), subsequent (established)
> > number of patients attending (visits per patient)
> > walk-in-clinic visits
> > accident and emergency visits
> > liaison consultations to other wards
> > cross-boundary flow;
> psychologists: similar information;
> domiciliary visits by consultants, CPNs, psychologists,
> > nurses, and others; number of cases receiving one or more visits;
> psychotherapy: number of new cases, cases carried, and
> > number of visits; number of group-therapy sessions and visits;
> day hospital: number of new cases/old patients per year,
> > number of attendances, number of patients carried;
> child psychiatry: as above;
> drug addiction: as above;
> residential services outside hospital: as per in-patient services;
> local-authority provision: hostels, day centres, psychiatric
> > social workers;
> voluntary-sector facilities: as per day and in-patient;
> private hospitals: in-patient and out-patient, as above.

A scheme for planning beds and resources

The following is how planners should determine the level of general psychiatric beds for a given catchment-area population for patients remaining in hospital up to 1 year.

(a) As a starting point, analyse current practice: the quantity of resources available per population and how these are used in the district.

(b) Determine the present bed resource as described in chapter 5; this is a reasonable and conservative place to begin. Calculate the current number of general psychiatry beds by discounting beds used for ESMI assessment, long-stay patients (in hospital more than 1 year), and non-district patients. Calculate the number of non-district patients in beds, as well as the numbers of beds in other units within the district which are supplementing the main acute-case service. The district will need to make a policy decision whether to allow for average cross-boundary inflow; this may require co-ordinated planning with other districts which may be taking the cross-boundary outflow. The working party found an average cross-boundary flow of 20% for the 40% of hospitals which had cross-boundary inflow; the remaining 60% of the sample had no inflow, but the working party did not determine if they had any cross-boundary outflow. Regional health authorities can provide data accounting for each districts' cross-boundary inflow and outflow.

(c) Make a decision which takes account of outflow to other units within the district and to other districts. If the service is to become locally 100% self-sufficient, local beds will have to be increased accordingly. Hospitals in some districts, such as those close to conurbations which do not have a nearby hospital, teaching hospital, etc., may wish to allow for cross-boundary inflow or outflow: this is one of many decisions which will determine the extent of resource spending.

(d) Calculate the true discharge rate for the catchment area, corresponding to the acute-case beds under review; this, as well as the activity analysis, can be used to determine if the beds are currently used efficiently. Local activity can be compared with that of hospitals in this report, and in due course, to nationally provided figures. Currently, Mental Health Enquiry figures are not broken down into acute-case, long-stay, ESMI, etc, categories.

(e) As a separate index, calculate the proportion of patients staying <1 week, <3 months, 3–6 months, 6–12 months, and more than 12 months. This can be used to check a major factor affecting bed need: the number and proportion of patients staying more than 3, 6, and 12 months. An indication of local performance can be obtained by a comparison with Table XIV. If there is a problem with too many EMSI, new long-stay patients, or patients staying more than 3 or 6 months in acute-case beds, this may need to be dealt with separately. However, plans must anticipate how these longer-stay patients are to be dealt with when planning for beds in the future, and must also be made to deal with the new long-stay patients, ESMI, and special client groups, e.g. young chronically ill and patients with alcohol-related morbidity.

(f) Calculate an *activity rating*. The working party's model can undoubtedly be improved on. However, whatever method is adopted, to be effective, the same method should be used widely for comparison purposes, and this in turn requires better book-keeping for each of the activity factors in all district services.

(g) Calculate the *social indices rating*, or Jarman Underprivileged Area score for the catchment area. Ideally, the National Census should be organised to provide social data for catchment areas, as their boundaries do not correspond to borough boundaries and National Census area borders.

(h) Calculate the total mental-health resource data for the service, using a model such as the one suggested above.

(i) Publish the social index data, activity data, number of discharged patients/bed and resource data, all adjusted for the size of population for all districts. Otherwise, districts will not be able to gauge their provision and use of resources relative to others, or estimate their needs. This recommendation will be partially satisfied by plans which flow from the Korner Report.

(j) Make allowance for the consequences of other plans which may affect the use of beds. For example, one district plans to phase out the use of beds for established long-stay patients by introducing 'wards' in the community: i.e. hostels in houses, with a high ratio of nurses to patients. It could be that acute exacerbations of illness, which in the past could be contained within the chronic-case hospital ward, will, under these conditions, require a short-term transfer to the acute-case DGH unit. This would demand a corresponding increase in the number of acute-case beds required to support chronically ill long-stay patients now transferred to the community. However, every planned change in the nature of the service will have to be carefully thought out in terms of its implications and consequences for the use of all other resources, including acute-case beds.

(k) Finally, starting from the median adjusted figure of 0.44 beds per 1000 population, and comparing this with the number of acute-case general psychiatric beds currently in use, take a decision to move from the present local bed figures either towards or away from the mean figures; this will depend on what decisions planners make to deal with the anomalies that this analysis shows up, and on how they plan to alter the way in which the resources are used and services deployed in the future.

Using this approach, planners will be in a much better position to make policy decisions. In some circumstances, it may be the best policy to provide a high level of service as a teaching and training resource and secondary referral centre. In other areas, there may be a disproportionate social need. In others, there may be a population which rejects psychiatric services, e.g. a tight-knit immigrant community or a closely knit industrial group, such as miners. Having made the analysis of current bed and resource use suggested here, planners should be in a position to make informed choices as to how these resources will be deployed.

9 Summary and conclusion

The working party has reviewed the relevant literature, carried out a comparison of eight psychiatric case registers, and completed an in-depth study of bed use and clinical practice in a stratified sample of 20 DGH-based psychiatric services, representing most regions in England. The purpose was to determine factors affecting bed needs for psychiatric patients, in order to provide an improved guideline for service planning. A greater than three-fold difference in acute-case bed/population ratios between districts (hypothesis 1) was confirmed. Next, as a starting figure for planning purposes, a median best estimate of 0.43–0.44 acute-case psychiatric beds (for patients staying less than 1 year) per 1000 population was determined for the non-demented adult population, after adjusting for cross-boundary flow and removing from the calculation hospitals which were clearly underresourced. This is a lower figure than the guideline of 0.5 beds per 1000, which had been adhered to until recently. However, it must be stressed that this is not a norm, but only the centre-point in a range of possible planning figures.

From a review of the literature, the working party found a consistent picture which showed a relationship between prevalence of psychiatric morbidity, uptake of resources, and social indices of poverty, deprivation, and socio-economic status. Moreover, in the districts studied, a relationship (hypothesis 2) which could be applied to planning was observed. Contrary to expectation (hypotheses 3 and 4), differences in the style of service and in the extent of ancillary hospital and social-service facilities and number of staff could not be shown to influence the variation in bed/population provision. The opposite tended to be the case: i.e. services with a high bed provision tended (with exceptions) to have more CPNs, more nurses, more day-hospital places, and a more active out-patient service (see Table XXIII). There was a close correlation between the number of consultants and the number of beds and also between the number of beds and number of discharges. It emerged that better-provided services had more beds, but also more of everything else; correspondingly, the services with the least beds tended to have the least of other resources.

Low bed ratios could not be explained by a more active community-based service with a different distribution of resources. This does not imply that alternative ways of working or the presence of better ancillary and community services are not relevant to the quality of the service. On the contrary, the picture is one of better services doing more per head of population and having more facilities, with worse services having fewer facilities, including beds, but this does not mean that high beds/population ratios are necessarily good. It is perfectly feasible to consider planning high-quality services which do not rely on many beds in some areas of the country, where the right conditions prevail, but this is likely to require the bed resources to be reallocated to a range of other resources, and not just the elimination of beds.

As suggested in this report, the investigation of current resource utilisation, compared with potential demand, will help planners decide if resources (not necessarily beds) should be increased or reduced. For example, an intensive increase in the community nursing service could lessen the need for beds. However, there is little reason to think that cutting beds without replacing them with other facilities will do other than reduce the service, which would then be reflected in a lower level of activity in relation to the social indices of potential demand. A different issue is where and whether better services are needed, because of greater morbidity and demand; the working party offered a way of assessing this.

Finally, the working party examined efficiency, in terms of the match between beds, resources, and the overall activity of the service, measured by the numbers of patient contacts at all levels of the service. In most services, beds are still the mainstay resource, limiting the extent to which demand from core morbidity can be met. The study of 400 consecutively discharged patients confirmed that the provision for longer-stay patients (requiring more than 6–12 months' hospitalisation) is a crucial factor affecting average length of stay (and bed throughput: the same thing) and, consequently, the number of acute-case beds required by the district. This confirms the prediction made by Hirsch (1983).

The approach to planning suggested here takes account of the working party's findings, but depends on there being better book-keeping and data-gathering by districts and regions, as well as reasoned, well-argued decision-making which takes account of local findings. An appraisal of the success of the service in meeting local demand, the views of social services, GPs, police, etc, as well as the size of waiting lists for out-patients, delays in admissions, and an appraisal of the economic resources available to invest in the service, will always remain part of the decision-making process. This report simply attempts to provide a method for making more informed judgements as to what should be done.

References

BAGLEY, C. (1973) Occupational class and symptoms of depression. *Social Science and Medicine*, **7**, 327–339.

BUGLASS, D., DUFFY, K. & KREITMAN, N. (1980) *A Register of Social and Medical Indices by Local Government Area in Edinburgh and Lothians.* Edinburgh: Scottish Office Central Research Papers.

BURKE, A. (1976) Attempted suicide among the Irish-born population of Birmingham. *British Journal of Psychiatry*, **128**, 534–537.

COCHRANE, R. (1977) Mental illness in immigrants to England and Wales: an analysis of mental hospital admissions 1971. *Social Psychiatry*, **12**, 25–35.

DOHRENWEND, B. S. & DOHRENWEND, B. P. (1975) Socio-cultural and social-psychological factors in the genesis of mental disorders. *Journal of Health and Social Behaviour*, **16**, 365–392.

DUNHAM, H. W. (1965) *Community and Psychiatry: an Epidemiological Analysis.* Detroit: Wayne State University Press.

FARIS, R. E. L. & DUNHAM, H. W. (1939) *Mental Disorders in Urban Areas.* Chicago: Hafner.

GIBBONS, J. L., JENNINGS, C. & WING, J. K. (1983) *Psychiatric Care in Eight Register Areas; Statistics from Eight Psychiatric Case Registers in Britain, 1976–81.* Southampton Psychiatric Case Register, Knowle Hospital, Fareham, Hants.

GOLDBERG, D. P. & HUXLEY, P. C. (1980) *Mental Illness in the Community. The Pathway to Psychiatric Care.* London: Tavistock Publications.

—— & MORRISON, S. L. (1963) Schizophrenia and social class. *British Journal of Psychiatry*, **109**, 785–802.

GOODMAN, A. B., SIEGEL, C., CRAIG, T. J. & LIN, S. P. (1983) The relationship between socio-economic class and prevalence of schizophrenia, alcoholism, and affective disorders treated by in-patient care in a suburban area. *American Journal of Psychiatry*, **140**, 166–170.

HIRSCH, S. R. (1983) Bed requirements for acute psychiatry units – the concept of a norm. *The Bulletin of the Royal College of Psychiatrists*, **7**, 118–122.

JARMAN, B. (1983) Identification of underprivileged areas. *British Medical Journal*, **286**, 1705–1709.

—— (1984) Validation and distribution of scores. *British Medical Journal*, **289**, 1587–1592.

KORNER REPORT (1982) *Steering Group on Health Services Information.* London: HMSO.

NUFFIELD/YORK PORTFOLIO SERIES. Folio No. 9, (1985) *Does Unemployment Kill?* London: Nuffield Provincial Hospital Trusts.

ODEGARD, O. (1983) Emigration and insanity: a study of mental disease among Norwegian-born population in Minnesota. *Acta Psychiatrica et Neurologica Scandinavica*, (suppl. 4).

PAYKEL, E. S. (1978) Meeting the needs of mental disorder – in the field of mental illness. *Health and Hygiene*, **1**, 193–196.

PLATT, S. & KREITMAN, N. (1985) Parasuicide and unemployment among men in Edinburgh – 1968–1982. *Psychological Medicine*, **15**, 113–123.

RESOURCE ALLOCATION WORKING PARTY (1976) *Sharing Resources for Health in England.* London: HMSO.

ROYAL COMMISSION ON THE NATIONAL HEALTH SERVICE (1979) *Report of the Royal Commission on the National Health Service.* London: HMSO.

Appendix 1

Jarman scales for estimating "predicted demand" for psychiatric services

The Jarman (1983, 1984) scores for all district health authorities are listed in descending order, ranked from the most underprivileged to the least under-privileged districts in the UK. Each variable was taken as a percentage of the resident population in the health district affected ('elderly alone', 'unskilled', etc.), except for 'unemployed', which was a percentage of the economically active population. The variables were then weighted according to the extent they were perceived in a GPs' survey to be contributing to GPs' workload. The score was then calculated as the weighted sum of these social variables normalised and standardised.

The weightings are shown below.

TABLE **XXIV**

Underprivileged areas: rank order of the weightings allocated by general practitioners to some common social factors (variables)

Variable	Weighting
Elderly living alone	6.62
*Older people (aged 65 and over)	6.19
*Children (aged under 5)	4.64
*Lower social classes (social class 5)	3.74
Poor housing (lacking amenities)	3.60
*Unemployment	3.34
Difficulties visiting	3.10
*Single-parent households	3.01
*Overcrowding of households	2.88
Non-married couple families	2.71
*Highly mobile people	2.68
*Ethnic minorities	2.50
Crime and vandalism	2.30

The variables marked * were used later in calculating the scores. The standard deviation for the district health authorities in England = 16.68.

TABLE XXV

List of district health authorities ranked in descending order from most to least underprivileged

DHA name	Residpop	Eldalone	Under5	Oneparnt	Unskilld	Unemplyd	Overcrdd	Movedhse	Ethnic	UPA8VARS	Rank
Tower Hamlets	139 996	6.32	6.95	3.81	10.75	15.57	21.55	11.74	20.28	54.89	1
Central Manchester	115 924	5.99	6.62	4.34	9.47	20.82	16.85	11.54	16.64	50.83	2
City & Hackney	184 230	5.90	6.86	5.11	7.28	15.00	18.25	10.60	27.45	48.62	3
Paddington & N Kensington	113 618	7.04	5.36	4.22	7.07	12.86	17.36	17.30	16.51	44.80	4
West Birmingham	209 907	5.07	7.29	3.38	7.83	19.70	20.43	9.21	30.14	44.46	5
Camberwell	213 864	5.96	6.11	5.02	7.58	12.64	13.07	12.14	21.86	39.97	6
West Lambeth	156 754	6.03	5.68	4.88	6.97	12.38	15.17	13.81	23.12	39.43	7
Islington	157 522	6.59	5.77	4.29	7.38	12.88	12.62	13.56	16.91	38.68	8
Bloomsbury	115 428	10.18	4.23	2.81	6.14	10.19	11.86	17.22	10.99	35.79	9
Bradford	328 952	5.66	7.66	2.70	6.76	13.48	14.91	10.77	14.08	35.75	10
North Manchester	143 779	6.94	6.30	3.23	8.25	17.39	13.01	9.42	4.04	35.01	11
Newham	209 128	5.15	7.15	3.00	7.81	12.68	18.11	9.17	26.60	34.84	12
Central Birmingham	177 271	5.72	6.77	2.94	5.79	16.44	15.88	10.55	20.09	33.83	13
Hammersmith and Fulham	144 616	7.01	5.11	3.80	6.45	11.10	14.72	13.46	15.27	31.76	14
Wandsworth	185 259	6.10	5.84	3.93	5.91	10.57	14.26	11.52	22.74	30.10	15
Lewisham & North Southwark	313 748	6.38	5.66	3.80	7.56	10.95	11.38	10.93	13.92	28.23	16
East Birmingham	203 881	5.24	6.69	2.38	6.67	16.71	16.78	7.73	15.83	24.91	17
Hampstead	98 517	7.61	4.88	3.56	3.62	10.73	9.94	16.63	10.00	24.68	18
Liverpool	503 721	5.72	5.92	2.82	8.69	19.83	11.96	8.49	1.68	22.89	19
Rochdale	211 003	5.46	7.08	2.85	6.50	12.87	11.00	9.10	5.11	22.32	20
Preston	124 414	6.06	6.29	2.42	6.52	12.88	11.43	9.51	9.01	21.03	21
Haringey	202 650	5.28	5.85	3.42	4.04	10.71	11.70	11.87	29.77	19.87	22
Oldham	219 461	5.90	6.59	2.84	6.41	11.06	9.58	9.07	5.07	18.77	23
Hull	312 621	5.64	6.45	2.46	8.57	14.62	8.61	9.54	0.73	18.68	24
Newcastle	272 913	6.56	5.67	2.61	6.72	14.15	9.79	10.19	2.42	18.67	25
Brent	251 238	4.51	6.20	3.05	4.25	10.09	17.17	10.71	33.48	18.67	26
Victoria	123 319	8.65	3.84	2.19	3.53	8.84	11.09	21.60	6.78	18.57	27
Burnley, Pendle & Rossendale	238 616	6.55	6.64	2.33	5.71	10.85	8.74	9.42	4.41	18.23	28
South Manchester	177 960	6.19	5.43	3.04	6.37	13.81	10.25	10.06	5.27	17.60	29
Dewsbury	161 740	5.70	6.89	2.08	5.34	10.94	12.26	9.36	8.22	17.31	30
Greenwich	209 873	5.54	6.49	3.21	5.70	9.62	8.73	10.26	7.97	17.25	31
Blackburn, Hyndburn & Ribble Valley	271 514	5.91	6.68	2.28	5.51	10.81	10.15	8.99	7.36	15.94	32
South Tees	299 483	4.30	6.85	2.46	8.04	17.85	9.51	8.52	1.98	14.96	33

Ealing	278 677	4.51	6.46	2.28	5.18	8.58	15.68	10.67	25.42	14.77	34
Milton Keynes	123 296	3.17	9.33	2.92	3.87	9.50	5.89	13.72	3.88	14.31	35
Wolverhampton	252 462	4.78	6.24	2.30	5.45	16.12	13.15	8.29	15.51	14.30	36
Salford	241 522	6.30	5.68	2.55	7.24	13.96	9.35	8.63	1.31	14.29	37
Calderdale	190 330	6.71	6.09	2.39	5.33	10.05	9.18	9.37	3.42	13.86	38
Bolton	260 228	5.73	6.51	2.25	6.02	11.60	9.76	8.39	6.44	13.84	39
Waltham Forest	214 595	5.88	6.33	2.73	4.29	8.85	11.07	7.97	17.48	13.23	40
Sunderland	294 102	4.95	6.63	2.45	6.13	16.67	9.23	9.43	0.56	12.97	41
Hartlepool	94 471	4.69	6.33	2.29	8.82	17.89	8.65	8.85	0.50	12.96	42
Coventry	310 216	4.77	6.23	2.66	5.34	15.21	12.19	8.36	9.61	12.67	43
Huddersfield	208 839	6.15	6.26	2.34	5.17	10.19	9.19	8.65	8.42	12.62	44
Sandwell	306 993	5.25	5.93	1.92	5.45	15.33	12.86	8.45	11.42	11.41	45
North West Durham	87 576	5.95	5.74	1.98	6.32	22.05	7.41	8.47	0.34	11.22	46
South Tyneside	160 100	6.01	5.58	2.32	7.34	16.77	9.76	7.63	0.63	11.19	47
South Birmingham	246 164	5.41	6.20	3.07	4.57	12.15	9.20	8.84	5.30	10.83	48
Leeds Eastern	344 103	5.62	5.95	2.80	5.39	11.10	8.36	9.46	4.99	10.25	49
St Helens & Knowsley	362 242	4.15	6.70	2.57	7.48	17.38	11.42	6.78	0.55	9.17	50
Tameside & Glossop	245 626	5.77	6.20	2.29	5.95	10.86	8.68	8.07	2.78	8.21	51
Gateshead	210 934	5.76	5.69	2.13	6.95	14.03	10.02	8.40	0.46	8.02	52
Hastings	149 353	9.48	4.90	2.20	3.06	8.61	4.14	10.82	1.54	7.18	53
Halton	140 541	3.90	7.37	2.46	6.08	12.88	7.63	9.51	0.58	6.80	54
South West Durham	155 931	5.27	6.14	2.13	6.55	13.72	8.11	9.03	0.35	6.73	55
Leeds Western	352 611	6.37	5.72	2.36	4.84	9.56	6.65	9.86	3.10	6.28	56
Brighton	286 077	8.64	4.81	2.20	3.17	8.72	6.00	11.20	2.24	5.96	57
North Tyneside	197 437	5.94	5.71	2.50	5.38	12.28	6.71	9.42	0.63	5.58	58
North Tees	171 891	4.08	6.98	2.23	6.06	15.15	7.00	8.65	1.40	5.23	59
Kettering	248 093	4.83	6.61	2.36	4.91	11.90	5.89	9.24	2.80	4.00	60
Airedale	171 655	6.29	6.15	2.01	4.95	7.54	5.80	9.51	2.86	3.80	61
Canterbury & Thanet	280 726	7.40	5.53	2.26	3.68	9.31	4.64	9.95	1.30	3.68	62
Lancaster	118 589	7.18	5.29	1.94	4.77	10.69	5.00	9.81	1.06	3.02	63
Peterborough	180 560	4.30	7.03	2.16	4.25	9.74	6.20	10.89	4.45	2.56	64
Sheffield	530 843	6.63	5.20	1.85	5.09	10.99	7.58	8.91	3.20	2.47	65
Wirral	358 832	5.48	6.09	2.37	5.06	13.03	5.60	8.08	0.74	1.84	66
Medway	315 963	4.22	7.44	2.00	4.86	8.87	6.33	9.22	3.39	1.49	67
Grimsby	159 852	4.75	6.19	2.11	6.43	11.27	6.74	9.05	0.73	0.86	68
Darlington	121 011	5.58	5.93	1.98	5.45	10.09	6.18	9.43	1.16	0.79	69

(*Continued*)

DHA name	Residpop	Eldalone	Under5	Oneparnt	Unskilld	Unemplyd	Overcrdd	Movedhse	Ethnic	UPA8VARS	Rank
Bristol & Weston	347 372	5.65	5.76	2.36	4.31	9.68	5.33	9.94	2.92	0.30	70
South Sefton	183 886	4.61	5.99	2.24	7.12	14.54	7.75	6.68	0.55	−0.02	71
Scunthorpe	191 881	4.37	6.32	1.88	6.86	13.41	5.36	8.92	1.13	−0.30	72
Plymouth	306 093	5.07	6.13	2.26	4.23	9.85	5.38	10.98	1.29	−0.72	73
Bury	175 452	5.43	6.27	2.12	4.70	8.96	6.55	8.03	2.12	−0.89	74
Wigan	307 723	5.14	6.36	1.95	5.73	11.25	6.70	7.25	0.47	−1.20	75
Southampton & SW Hampshire	394 781	5.16	5.94	2.08	5.33	8.00	5.87	9.97	2.80	−1.63	76
Leicestershire	835 647	4.61	6.55	1.96	3.78	8.35	7.65	9.10	8.52	−1.83	77
Nottingham	594 794	5.18	5.88	2.40	3.82	9.24	7.18	9.01	4.47	−1.94	78
Durham	234 363	5.10	6.18	1.94	4.55	10.78	7.56	9.18	0.35	−1.99	79
South Bedfordshire	269 325	3.50	7.48	2.14	3.23	8.54	9.04	9.16	9.20	−2.02	80
Walsall	265 922	4.24	6.16	1.85	4.15	13.59	10.57	7.80	7.17	−2.06	81
West Cumbria	136 835	4.77	6.07	1.78	7.13	10.76	6.70	8.57	0.31	−2.18	82
Swindon	212 624	4.04	6.71	1.96	4.44	8.53	5.99	11.93	2.51	−2.71	83
Great Yarmouth & Waveney	185 380	6.02	5.68	1.86	5.28	10.16	3.98	9.01	0.74	−2.79	84
Isle of Wight	114 878	7.14	5.03	1.94	3.70	9.88	3.91	10.50	0.80	−2.89	85
Doncaster	286 924	4.50	6.30	2.19	3.99	12.03	6.79	9.46	1.24	−3.00	86
Worthing	229 950	9.38	4.92	1.68	2.37	5.88	3.67	9.67	1.53	−3.19	87
Richmond, Twickenham & Roehampton	224 285	6.48	5.06	2.47	2.69	6.37	6.62	10.92	5.58	−3.38	88
Scarborough	136 311	7.12	5.10	1.69	4.89	9.22	4.44	9.19	0.47	−3.45	89
Hounslow & Spelthorne	290 970	4.55	5.98	2.06	3.95	6.30	9.75	9.65	12.56	−3.47	90
Northampton	276 874	4.56	6.85	2.21	3.53	7.04	4.98	10.38	3.10	−3.88	91
Rotherham	250 359	4.47	6.41	2.00	4.39	11.58	7.53	8.18	1.36	−4.15	92
Portsmouth & SE Hampshire	495 446	4.96	6.11	2.25	3.48	7.82	4.93	11.77	1.96	−4.16	93
Southern Derbyshire	515 475	5.09	6.07	1.83	5.17	7.77	6.38	8.51	3.93	−4.22	94
Cornwall & Isles of Scilly	418 625	5.71	5.68	1.88	3.63	11.34	4.82	10.33	0.79	−4.23	95
Wakefield	140 858	5.13	6.34	2.21	3.75	7.20	6.68	9.08	1.74	−4.26	96
North East Essex	274 672	6.27	5.94	1.86	3.51	7.39	3.93	9.93	1.51	−4.43	97
Basildon and Thurrock	278 309	3.50	7.02	2.41	5.73	9.30	6.09	8.28	1.88	−4.47	98
South East Kent	248 931	6.23	5.76	1.87	3.01	7.98	4.96	10.50	1.44	−4.61	99
North Lincolnshire	258 488	5.08	6.14	1.84	3.62	9.26	4.97	11.59	0.88	−4.73	100
Torbay	217 945	7.52	4.69	1.95	3.14	10.36	4.01	9.98	0.94	−4.95	101
Northumberland	295 451	5.37	6.22	1.68	4.36	8.36	5.70	9.54	0.40	−5.34	102
West Norfolk & Wisbech	173 884	5.34	5.94	1.72	4.22	10.55	5.26	9.56	0.72	−5.47	103

Enfield	257 154	5.39	5.82	1.95	3.25	6.59	7.11	8.23	14.03	−5.54	104
Blackpool, Wyre & Fylde	311 065	7.33	4.63	1.88	3.87	9.76	4.66	9.60	0.62	−5.71	105
North Staffordshire	462 207	5.17	5.86	1.72	5.44	10.40	7.36	7.19	1.35	−5.71	106
East Suffolk	302 188	5.42	6.28	1.60	4.54	6.43	4.46	10.06	1.82	−5.79	107
Chester	176 375	4.39	5.86	2.25	5.73	10.86	6.25	8.45	0.84	−6.02	108
Croydon	316 306	4.54	6.04	2.44	2.77	6.15	7.75	9.83	12.04	−6.08	109
West Suffolk	209 010	4.40	6.83	1.92	3.57	6.48	4.76	12.06	1.19	−6.15	110
Shropshire	370 355	4.57	6.28	1.88	4.20	9.93	5.21	9.92	1.36	−6.29	111
East Cumbria	170 795	5.58	5.66	1.76	5.48	7.92	5.79	8.69	0.45	−6.71	112
Eastbourne	205 585	8.42	4.89	1.75	2.56	5.73	3.11	10.31	1.58	−6.75	113
Barnet	290 197	5.28	5.82	1.90	2.04	6.22	8.07	10.22	12.81	−6.97	114
West Lancashire	106 385	3.82	6.65	2.49	3.61	11.89	5.44	9.12	0.74	−7.09	115
Trafford	221 002	5.26	5.73	2.19	3.83	8.78	6.05	7.83	3.86	−7.29	116
East Dorset	401 468	7.15	4.83	1.74	2.96	8.16	4.09	11.10	1.15	−7.62	117
Warrington	168 826	4.63	6.37	1.79	4.83	9.40	5.82	7.88	0.86	−8.05	118
Pontefract	169 028	4.74	5.84	2.07	3.98	9.94	7.87	8.85	0.43	−8.06	119
North Bedfordshire	232 839	3.99	7.02	1.77	3.90	5.96	5.37	9.93	5.47	−8.16	120
West Dorset	177 516	6.33	5.44	1.71	3.26	6.87	3.91	11.15	1.05	−8.31	121
Merton & Sutton	332 649	5.79	5.63	1.99	2.99	5.32	5.98	9.16	7.21	−8.40	122
Oxfordshire	473 957	4.12	6.50	1.81	3.82	6.54	5.19	12.10	2.58	−8.52	123
Bromsgrove & Redditch	153 373	3.50	7.51	2.35	2.78	9.03	4.62	9.38	2.09	−8.59	124
Hillingdon	226 263	4.53	6.10	1.94	3.87	5.67	7.45	9.16	6.63	−9.05	125
Barnsley	223 903	5.04	5.86	1.79	3.88	10.48	8.12	7.73	0.37	−9.08	126
Cambridge	246 756	5.15	6.15	1.84	3.64	5.39	3.86	11.33	1.84	−9.14	127
South Cumbria	164 066	6.14	5.33	1.87	4.51	7.32	4.46	8.79	0.45	−9.34	128
Exeter	280 717	6.40	5.31	1.85	3.03	7.13	4.31	10.18	1.03	−9.41	129
Chichester	162 216	7.19	4.98	1.63	2.98	6.75	3.60	10.54	1.32	−9.58	130
Huntingdon	112 216	3.53	7.45	1.90	3.05	6.29	4.33	12.17	1.68	−9.65	131
South East Staffordshire	246 846	3.65	7.05	1.79	4.22	9.16	5.66	8.47	1.88	−10.00	132
Southmead	220 632	4.88	5.85	2.10	3.47	7.46	4.62	9.96	2.48	−10.17	133
Salisbury	117 653	5.46	5.74	1.57	3.37	6.26	4.82	11.40	1.58	−10.38	134
South Lincolnshire	284 454	5.21	5.85	1.53	4.13	8.62	4.56	9.72	0.72	−10.50	135
Bassetlaw	101 120	4.62	5.96	1.85	4.24	8.86	6.08	9.01	0.67	−10.61	136
North Birmingham	159 146	4.94	5.15	2.02	3.52	11.19	6.55	8.63	4.38	−10.68	137
Chorley and South Ribble	187 546	4.28	6.77	1.86	3.94	7.42	5.30	8.46	0.90	−10.83	138
Southend	314 280	5.63	5.97	1.95	2.71	7.40	4.25	8.71	1.63	−10.88	139

(Continued)

DHA name	Residpop	Eldalone	Under5	Oneparnt	Unskilld	Unemplyd	Overcrdd	Movedhse	Ethnic	UPA8VARS	Rank
Cheltenham & District	197 239	5.68	5.62	2.02	2.84	6.20	4.64	10.21	1.53	−10.99	140
Stockport	288 982	5.26	5.99	2.06	3.08	8.00	5.20	7.94	1.48	−11.03	141
Norwich	435 263	5.66	5.59	1.89	3.48	7.46	3.64	9.84	0.85	−11.18	142
Northallerton	103 701	4.76	6.14	1.51	3.50	6.57	3.73	12.83	0.80	−11.40	143
East Berkshire	344 333	3.87	6.57	1.74	2.92	5.75	7.51	10.23	7.98	−11.46	144
Central Nottinghamshire	280 834	4.76	6.21	1.81	3.64	7.60	6.22	8.50	0.70	−11.65	145
Worcester & District	224 971	4.92	6.01	1.80	3.93	8.15	4.48	8.80	1.03	−11.67	146
Aylesbury Vale	130 771	3.85	6.93	1.63	3.36	5.26	5.06	11.55	3.41	−11.72	147
North Hertfordshire	180 547	4.08	6.45	2.12	3.05	7.80	5.13	8.99	4.50	−11.74	148
Bath	371 113	5.27	5.83	1.86	3.28	6.38	4.44	9.95	1.56	−11.95	149
Crewe	241 872	4.75	6.09	1.59	4.47	8.46	5.69	7.85	0.84	−12.30	150
Somerset	368 980	5.58	5.71	1.78	3.51	6.47	3.82	9.67	0.95	−12.32	151
Gloucester	295 927	4.71	6.00	1.73	3.85	7.51	5.70	8.67	2.20	−12.35	152
Harrogate	126 344	6.23	5.41	1.71	3.01	5.53	3.17	11.09	0.93	−12.41	153
Dartford & Gravesham	221 036	4.00	6.46	1.72	4.47	7.21	5.77	7.86	4.54	−12.59	154
York	240 691	5.19	5.66	1.73	4.28	6.12	4.65	9.77	0.79	−12.82	155
North Warwickshire	172 600	3.81	6.31	1.77	4.16	10.70	6.97	7.46	2.17	−12.84	156
Barking, Havering & Brentwood	460 702	4.60	5.75	1.94	4.58	7.11	7.89	6.85	2.81	−13.00	157
Herefordshire	146 870	4.85	5.80	1.69	3.77	7.59	5.55	9.71	0.65	−13.08	158
Kidderminster & District	99 179	4.53	6.23	1.87	3.42	10.20	4.99	7.43	1.09	−13.13	159
Harrow	196 159	4.77	5.93	1.62	2.15	5.41	7.87	8.75	15.28	−13.17	160
Redbridge	224 731	5.01	5.65	1.77	2.98	6.58	6.88	7.41	11.22	−13.21	161
North Devon	123 290	5.71	5.33	1.68	3.17	7.86	4.12	9.96	0.75	−13.70	162
Rugby	84 686	4.39	6.08	1.96	2.80	7.28	5.68	8.69	4.82	−14.06	163
North Derbyshire	357 773	5.28	5.67	1.54	4.35	7.53	5.25	7.93	0.51	−14.22	164
Dudley	298 524	4.55	5.97	1.47	3.47	10.78	6.58	6.70	3.43	−14.62	165
West Berkshire	396 947	4.05	6.38	1.78	2.75	5.25	5.63	10.95	3.76	−14.89	166
Southport & Formby	114 318	6.62	5.03	1.66	2.69	8.62	2.81	8.75	0.81	−15.17	167
Mid Downs	257 956	4.18	6.61	1.66	3.30	4.55	3.82	10.54	2.88	−15.57	168
Basingstoke & N Hampshire	198 601	3.49	6.93	1.87	3.28	5.23	4.59	10.66	2.13	−15.58	169
Winchester	196 989	4.53	6.12	1.59	3.09	4.72	3.86	11.94	1.81	−16.05	170
Kingston & Esher	177 924	5.66	5.53	1.78	2.01	4.78	4.40	9.95	4.76	−16.18	171
South Warwickshire	212 515	4.62	5.65	1.76	3.07	6.81	5.29	9.05	3.37	−17.05	172
Mid Essex	266 462	3.96	6.93	1.64	3.10	5.11	3.71	9.28	1.61	−17.70	173

Residpop	eldalone	under5	oneparnt	unskilld	unemplyd	overcrdd	movedhse	ethnic	UPA8VARS	
Maidstone	186 947	4.17	6.48	1.59	2.97	6.15	5.02	9.01	1.60	−17.73	174
Bexley	214 355	4.45	5.82	1.73	3.62	5.64	5.13	7.81	4.18	−18.71	175
Tunbridge Wells	194 711	5.55	5.51	1.51	2.95	5.01	4.10	9.03	1.61	−18.89	176
South West Hertfordshire	239 010	4.51	5.82	1.78	3.02	5.22	5.14	8.43	3.93	−19.26	177
West Essex	256 224	4.06	5.98	1.89	3.20	6.36	5.23	8.61	1.99	−19.34	178
North West Surrey	200 930	4.50	5.84	1.68	2.62	4.50	4.99	10.27	3.00	−19.66	179
Frenchay	211 062	4.44	6.17	1.72	3.08	6.00	4.04	8.03	1.80	−19.74	180
South West Surrey	173 779	5.33	5.60	1.61	2.26	4.15	3.71	10.42	2.07	−20.14	181
West Surrey & NE Hampshire	265 009	3.31	6.83	1.74	2.16	4.35	4.11	12.52	2.75	−20.31	182
Bromley	294 526	4.96	5.36	1.87	2.47	5.23	4.82	8.93	3.60	−20.55	183
North West Hertfordshire	252 882	4.11	6.26	1.78	2.34	5.34	4.34	9.30	2.93	−20.69	184
Macclesfield	174 128	5.02	5.55	1.67	3.19	6.65	3.65	8.20	0.84	−20.70	185
Solihull	197 933	3.73	5.74	2.53	2.37	9.04	5.99	7.54	1.86	−20.79	186
Mid Staffordshire	296 588	3.57	6.27	1.59	3.34	8.30	5.73	8.16	1.09	−20.96	187
East Yorkshire	178 911	5.49	5.17	1.46	3.08	6.78	3.48	9.08	0.59	−21.26	188
East Surrey	183 797	5.10	5.49	1.46	2.42	4.31	4.34	9.56	2.18	−22.89	189
Wycombe	271 006	3.79	6.19	1.56	2.07	4.60	5.05	9.46	4.75	−24.49	190
East Hertfordshire	278 321	3.84	5.98	1.61	2.86	4.99	4.25	8.40	1.79	−26.59	191
Mid Surrey	166 875	4.98	5.16	1.35	1.68	3.77	3.25	8.54	2.42	−32.79	192

Residpop=resident population; eldalone=elderly people living alone; under5=children aged under 5; oneparnt=single-parent households; unskilld=unskilled workers; unemplyd=unemployed people; overcrdd=overcrowded households; movedhse=people who had moved house; ethnic=ethnic minorities; UPA8VARS=people from underprivileged area – eight variables.

Appendix 2

Components of a comprehensive psychiatric service

The following are lists of the component parts of an idealised service for the mentally ill in a community. Some of the headings refer to structural components, such as beds, day places, workshops, centres, housing; and others to services, such as psychiatric teams, specialist departments, community psychiatric nursing services, out-patient clinics and domiciliary services, rehabilitation teams, crisis intervention programmes, i.e. the manpower or staffing components. A further part refers to the necessary organisational arrangements for the co-ordination and management of services.

The lists are divided into sections, based on groups of patients who appear to need separated services, though there is bound to be overlap and joint use. The lists are constructed against the background of the use of beds, especially admission beds in general-hospital psychiatric units. It is suggested that the presence or absence of all the other elements of the service will in some way affect the free movement of patients in and out of the psychiatric admission unit, and therefore determine the numbers of beds used and staff required.

Summary of sections: general psychiatry; psychiatry of chronic mental illness; psychiatry of old age; alcoholism; drug dependency; forensic psychiatry; psychiatry of disturbed behaviour; psychiatry of adolescence; psychiatry of childhood; psychiatry in primary health care; psychiatry within social services; and
Organisational arrangements for: planning, management, co-ordination with other services, and monitoring.

General psychiatry

In-patient beds
Locally based in DGH or general hospital with access to the whole range of general medical services and investigation (especially special neurological and neurosurgical investigation)
Out-patient clinics
Within reasonable travelling distance of community served

Walk-in or emergency clinics
  Daily, if not at night and weekends
Psychiatric service for accident and emergency departments
Liaison psychiatry
  For other departments including self-injury and self-poisoning
Day hospital places
   (i) In association with the main in-patient unit
   (ii) Peripheral day-hospital units within reasonable travelling distance of community served
   (iii) Intermittent day-hospital places for small or scattered population
   (iv) Specialist day-hospital places, e.g., for alcoholism, elderly mentally infirm, children, adolescents
Community psychiatric teams
  Consultant-led multidisciplinary teams responsible for an agreed catchment area
Sheltered housing (warden supervised)
Very sheltered housing (warden supervised and augmented home care services)
Independent housing: special housing schemes and housing associations
Day hospitals: special arrangements for chronic mental illness
Day centres: provided by Local Authority
Occupation and activities centres: provided by voluntary bodies, e.g., MIND
Luncheon and social clubs: provided by local authority
Sheltered work: (i) Local Authority; (ii) voluntary bodies, e.g., PRA; (iii) Department of Employment; (iv) IRUs; (v) Industrial Therapy Organisations; and (vi) enclave working
Social Services Area Teams
  Either generic social work for a defined population ('patch') or specialist social work arranged in client groups
District physiotherapy services
  Working within hospital and community services but especially for the elderly frail and mentally infirm
Secure accommodation
   (i) Within the general psychiatric service
   (ii) Access to medium secure accommodation (see also forensic psychiatry)
Non-acute hospital services
  Continuing care wards (residential, long-stay, slow stream rehabilitation)
  Rehabilitation places
  Intensive care unit – disturbed ward, behaviour-modification ward, token economy ward
Mother and baby unit
  May be within psychiatric unit or a unit for mothers and young children

Psychiatry of chronic mental illness

Rehabilitation and resettlement team
Social services area teams
  either generic social work for a defined local population or specialist social work arranged in client groups
Occupational therapy department with ADL
Hospital rehabilitation unit or wards

Progressive hospital accommodation
  cubicles, single rooms, group living, flats, rehabilitation homes within hospitals
Day hospitals
  special arrangements for chronic mental illness
Day centres
  provided by local authority
Local-authority old persons' homes
Sheltered lodging scheme
  landlady groups
Supervised accommodation
    (i) jointly with housing department
    (ii) housing allocation for mentally ill people
Staff grouped homes
Group homes
    (i) run by district council
    (ii) run by voluntary associations, e.g. MIND, housing associations
Halfway homes, run by, e.g. Richmond Fellowship, etc.
Hospital hostels
  the experimental schemes
Mental-illness hostels
    (i) residential
    (ii) assessment and crisis
    (iii) rehabilitation
Special hostels
  run by, e.g. St Dismas, the Cyrenians
Rehabilitation houses
Sheltered housing
  warden-supervised
Very sheltered housing
    (i) warden-supervised and with augmented home-care services
    (ii) managed jointly by social services and housing departments
Independent housing
  special housing schemes and housing associations
Industrial therapy (graded work)
Sheltered work
    (i) local authority
    (ii) voluntary bodies, e.g. Psychiatric Rehabilitation Association
    (iii) Department of Employment
    (iv) industrial rehabilitation units
    (v) enclave working
Social rehabilitation groups – literacy, social skills, domestic management
Joint health and social-services resettlement scheme

Psychiatry of old age

A department of psychogeriatrics or mental health care of the elderly
Psychogeriatric assessment unit
  Access to geriatric and general hospital departments
Unit for treatment of functional psychiatric illness

Joint assessment between psychiatry and geriatric departments
  A ward or shared beds
Fast-stream rehabilitation beds
  Special contribution from OT, physiotherapy, and psychology
Slow-stream rehabilitation beds
Continuing-care beds
  Sick ward and nursing of infirmity
Holiday-relief beds
Intermittent-care beds
  Care sharing '10 in a bed'
Crisis and emergency beds
Day-hospital places
  For elderly mentally infirm, especially for assessment and relief of supporters
Out-patient clinics
  Referrals other than in crisis
Domiciliary consultation and assessment
  In crisis and to plan management
Consultation, advisory and support services
  For general practice, residential homes and social workers on elderly mentally
  infirm
Day centres for elderly mentally ill
Specialist community team
  for elderly mentally ill, especially specialist CPNs
Relative support groups
Retired-person's advisory group
  Network for information and counselling
Home-help services
Community nursing services
Health visitors
Home meals
Street wardens and neighbourhood schemes
Home-care assistants
Augmented home care ('flying squad')
Elderly persons homes
    (i) Special EMSI homes
    (ii) EMSI wings in ordinary homes
    (iii) Group living ordinary homes
The private sector for old people
    (i) Rest homes
    (ii) Nursing homes
    (iii) Housing associations

Alcoholism

 Special interest consultant
 Alcoholism unit, out-patients and day hospital
 Detoxification beds or arrangements
 Access to regional unit

Information and counselling service
  preferably through a Council for Alcoholism
A forum for interested agencies
  Health and Social Services, probation, police, magistrates, prisons, industry,
  GPs, church, hostels, etc.
Self-help groups
  AA, Al-Anon, Al-ateens, ACCEPT, Libra Project, etc.
Half-way house
  recovering alcoholics
Hostels for persistent drinkers
  St Dismas, Cyrenians, etc.
Service to hostels
  Church Army, reception centres, etc.

Drug dependency

Consultant with special responsibility
Other professional staff
Drug-addiction clinics
In-patient beds for withdrawal
Advisory and counselling service to other agencies
Self-help and support groups
Special hostels or treatment centres

Forensic psychiatry

Consultant with responsibility
Medium secure unit
Specialist team
Out-patient clinics
Half-way houses
Supervised accommodation
Employment
Access to services for chronic mental illness
Contacts with special hospitals, prison, remand centres, probation service, etc.

Psychiatry of disturbed behaviour

Consultant with responsibility within the district
Beds for treating disturbed patients
  Special ward: disturbed ward, intensive-care unit
Access to forensic and psychology services

Psychiatry of adolescence

In-patient unit
  Needs to cover whole range of cases, including disturbed psychotic adolescents,
  those with aggressive and destructive behaviour as well as those requiring
  psychotherapy

Out-patient clinics
Therapy services
Schooling
Residential care
Local-authority homes for observation and assessment
Local-authority fostering schemes
Advisory service to other agencies

Psychiatry of childhood

Services are not likely to have much impact on adult services, except where there is difficulty in placing a psychotic child, or where staffing of child guidance or child psychiatry is seriously depleted.

Psychiatry in primary health care

Availability of specialist advice
Postgraduate education
Consultant availability in health centres and surgeries
   For advice, discussion and consultation (e.g. Balint groups)
Contribution of CPNs
Early and easy referral systems
Joint working
   Between primary health care, social-work teams and psychiatric teams
Crisis and community intervention schemes (*see also* General psychiatry)

Psychiatry within social services

Joint working with shared population
   Shared management plans
Means of communication and sharing of knowledge and resources
Specialist advice available at times of crisis
   (i) Use of Mental Health Act
   (ii) Doctors approved under Section 12
Follow-up and continuity before and after specialist treatment
Family management
Support for treatment and casework

Organisational arrangements

Planning
A joint strategic plan for mental-health services agreed between the health authority and the social-services department of the Local Authority in the Joint Consultative Committee.
Co-ordination by the joint health care planning team through a subgroup for mental-health services, advised by a psychiatric division. A less satisfactory alternative is the combination of the plans of the district mental-health care planning team and the mental-health development group (or equivalent) of the social-services department.

Management
   A psychiatric-services management team, including administration, finance and
   social services as well as clinical disciplines (Nodder Report) or a mental-illness
   management unit responsible for service management.
   Hospital management teams responsible for day-to-day management of
   component hospitals.
   Clinical teams: departmental, unit and ward management.

Evaluation of monitoring
   Monitoring of objectives by panel of health-authority members
   Monitoring of objectives by PSMT and clinical teams
   Medical audit of clinical performance
   Regular statistical bulletin
   Annual reports
   Monitoring by CHC
   External evaluation
      By health advisory service (service performance), Royal College of Psychiatrists
      (training), and GNC (nurse training).

Appendix 3

Use of Jarman Underprivileged Area score to weight district resource allocation and bed requirements within regional health authorities

Regions presently allocate acute-case mental-health resources solely on the basis of district population size, by prescribing a set allocation of resource provision. For example, several regions have chosen a level of bed provision of 0.35 beds per 1000 population for acute-case psychiatric services. However, as we have shown, there is a strong association between the socio-demographic characteristics of an area and both the level of psychiatric morbidity and demand for psychiatric services within it. Socio-demographic indices, such as the Jarman Underprivileged Area score (UPA score), have been shown in this report to be highly predictive of psychiatric admission rates (see the literature review in chapter 2 of this report). Acute-case psychiatric admissions and the resources required to fund alternatives to hospital-based treatment account for the major part of acute-case psychiatric service expenditure in most DGH- and mental-hospital-based services. It follows that it would be valid to weight both acute-case psychiatric-service bed provision and total expenditure according to socio-demographic indices. Such an approach would be a considerable improvement on the present method, which distributes regional resources solely on a per-unit-population basis. We have chosen to use the socio-demographic characteristics of a population for weighting the level of service provision, rather than admission rates themselves, because they are independent of local-service factors (admission policy, availability of beds, teaching-hospital practice, etc.) which affect admission rates. This method is also suitable when a new service is being set up that might differ in character from the previous one (new hospital, new catchment area, etc.).

For the purpose of this example, we shall use the North West Thames Regional Health Authority data already discussed in this report (chapter 2 and Table XXIII). In brief, for 1984, the district of residence adult psychiatric admission rates for all patients, and for those under 65 years old, correlate very closely with the UPA score, $r_s = 0.76$ and $r_s = 0.80$, respectively.

Bed requirements

The relationship between admission rates and UPA score can be expressed mathematically as:

$$Y = a + bX$$

where Y is the predicted admission rate within a region for a given value of X; the UPA score, b, is the slope of the regression line of admission rates against UPA score; and a is the intercept for that line (the value of Y when $x = 0$). The relationship is illustrated graphically in Fig. 7, p. 55, which shows admission rates for the under-65-year-olds, because services for the over-65s tend to be dealt with separately. The values of UPA scores are readily available for each district in England. District admission rates are presently available from the Mental Health Enquiry, and will soon be available as Korner data. The constant b can be calculated by a number of methods (we used the method of least squares) and the intercept, a, can be calculated once b is known.

To predict bed requirements, a region must set a target for a regional average level of bed provision, such as the 0.35 beds per 1000 population set by the North West Thames Regional Health Authority. This is the level of bed provision a region would provide for a district with the average (mean) UPA score for health districts in the region. Assuming that bed requirements are proportional to admission rates, we can predict the district bed requirements per 1000 of the population by the equation:

$$\text{PBD A} = \text{RTA} \times \frac{\text{PAR A}}{\text{PAR R}}$$

PBD A is the predicted beds per 1000 of the population for district A.
RTA is the regional target average.
PAR A is the predicted admission rate for district A.
PAR R is the predicted admission rate a district would have if it had a UPA score at the mean for its region.
$\dfrac{\text{PAR A}}{\text{PAR R}}$ is the factor for weighting resources for district A.

Example

A district is about to set up its own DGH psychiatric service in the North West Thames Regional Health Authority. It has a UPA score of plus 20, the RTA is 0.35 beds per 1000 population, and the population is 150 000. The mean regional UPA score is plus 0.5. Using the regional data in Table XXII, values of a = 2.94 and b = 0.045 were calculated by the method of least squares for the equation $Y = a + bX$.

$$\text{PAR A} = a + (b \times \text{UPA A})$$
$$\text{PAR A} = 2.94 + (0.045 \times 20)$$
$$= 3.84 \text{ admissions per 1000 population per year}$$

$$\text{PAR R} = a + (b \times \text{UPA R})$$
$$= 2.94 + (0.045 \times 0.5)$$
$$= 2.96 \text{ admissions per 1000 population per year}$$

$$\text{PBD A} = \text{RTA} \times \frac{\text{PAR A}}{\text{PAR R}} = \text{RTA} \times \frac{\text{PAR A}}{\text{PAR R}}$$

$$= 0.35 \times \frac{3.84}{2.96}$$

$$= 0.45 \text{ beds per 1000 population}$$

For a catchment area of 150 000 and a PBD A of 0.45 beds per 1000 population, the district mental-health unit would have a predicted bed requirement of 68 acute-case beds.

The weighting factor for the district is:

$$\frac{\text{PAR A}}{\text{PAR R}} = 1.3$$

Determining the financial grant for a district's mental-health service

In many regions, a figure is set for regional spending on psychiatric services. This is then divided by the number in the regional population to give a *per capita* value, and is multiplied by the population size of a district to estimate the grant for each district. It can be argued that the financial grant should be adjusted to take into account differences in psychiatric morbidity (the principle of the Resource Allocation Working Party) rather than just the size of the population. We could argue that, in general, acute-case admission rates are the best indicators of the extent of the psychiatric morbidity in a district that depends on hospital-based services. Where services have shifted from a hospital- to a community-based service, it should be possible to identify the equivalent of an admitted patient, i.e. severely disturbed patients requiring high-dependency services, albeit in the community. The high correlation of UPA score and admission rates enables one to calculate a morbidity weighting factor, which can be taken into account in adjusting the financial allocation available for psychiatric services.

We have not studied the use of chronic-case psychiatric services and their relationship to socio-demographic factors, but it would seem to be a reasonable working assumption that the needs of the chronically mentally ill will be related to the overall demand for acute-case psychiatric services, and to the same social characteristics which predict them. Thus the morbidity weighting suggested here for acute-case services could be reasonably applied to the total mental-health service grant. However, districts with a changed or changing population size would have acquired most of their long-stay patients in the past at a rate appropriate to the district's previous population size. Furthermore, in the past, the large mental hospitals have often had large catchment areas covering a number of districts. This has led to some districts in which large hospitals are so sited that they have responsibility for many long-stay patients not originating from that district, and other districts having responsibility for very few long-stay patients. Where there is an accumulated established long-stay population, another approach is to identify the number of chronically mentally ill in long-term hospital and community accommodation, and calculate a separate grant on a *per capita* basis; however, this has the danger of depending on declared cases, overlooking those who should have a service but have slipped through the net. More research is needed, but we would recommend that both approaches be used to inform planners of the needs of the chronically mentally ill in and out of hospital.

To adjust district budgets, one would simply apply the resource weighting factors derived from regional admission data and UPA scores as described in the 'Bed requirements' section above to the regional target *per capita* budget. For example, the district in the example above would have the regional target *per capita* budget multiplied by its predicted admission rate and divided by the regional predicted average admission rate, i.e. its budget would be multiplied by a factor of 1.3.

It should be understood that the Jarman UPA score was chosen for practical rather than theoretical reasons. It was the only socio-demographic index readily available for health districts, and it may be superseded by another similar index in the future. However, it was found to correlate highly with admission rates, both within the district of South Hammersmith and Fulham, and across the North West Thames Region (see the literature review in chapter 2 of this report).